AF745194

Chronic Kidney Disease - New Updates

Edited by Henry H.L. Wu

Published in London, United Kingdom

Chronic Kidney Disease - New Updates
http://dx.doi.org/10.5772/intechopen.1008028
Edited by Henry H.L. Wu

Contributors
Crystal Ayazo, George Metry, Haerani Rasyid, Idopise Umana, Jun Mochizuki, Katsuhiko Fukuda, Maura Andini Setiabudi, Nivedha Balaji, Qi Guo, Shaw Watanabe, Shimaa Shabaka, Shu Wakino, Tan Wei, Trianingsih, Wen Wen, Yasushi Saiga, Yunanto Kurnia

© The Editor(s) and the Author(s) 2025

The rights of the editor(s) and the author(s) have been asserted in accordance with the Copyright, Designs and Patents Act 1988. All rights to the book as a whole are reserved by INTECHOPEN LIMITED. The book as a whole (compilation) cannot be reproduced, distributed or used for commercial or non-commercial purposes without INTECHOPEN LIMITED's written permission. Enquiries concerning the use of the book should be directed to INTECHOPEN LIMITED rights and permissions department (permissions@intechopen.com).

Violations are liable to prosecution under the governing Copyright Law.

(cc) BY

Individual chapters of this publication are distributed under the terms of the Creative Commons Attribution 4.0 License which permits commercial use, distribution and reproduction of the individual chapters, provided the original author(s) and source publication are appropriately acknowledged. If so indicated, certain images may not be included under the Creative Commons license. In such cases users will need to obtain permission from the license holder to reproduce the material. More details and guidelines concerning content reuse and adaptation can be found at http://www.intechopen.com/copyright-policy.html.

Notice

Statements and opinions expressed in the chapters are these of the individual contributors and not necessarily those of the editors or publisher. No responsibility is accepted for the accuracy of information contained in the published chapters. The publisher assumes no responsibility for any damage or injury to persons or property arising out of the use of any materials, instructions, methods or ideas contained in the book.

First published in London, United Kingdom, 2025 by IntechOpen
IntechOpen is the global imprint of INTECHOPEN LIMITED, registered in England and Wales, registration number: 11086078, 167-169 Great Portland Street, London, W1W 5PF, United Kingdom

For EU product safety concerns: IN TECH d.o.o., Prolaz Marije Krucifikse Kozulić 3, 51000 Rijeka, Croatia, info@intechopen.com or visit our website at intechopen.com.

British Library Cataloguing-in-Publication Data
A catalogue record for this book is available from the British Library

Chronic Kidney Disease - New Updates
Edited by Henry H.L. Wu
p. cm.
Print ISBN 978-1-83635-328-7
Online ISBN 978-1-83635-327-0
eBook (PDF) ISBN 978-1-83635-329-4

If disposing of this product, please recycle the paper responsibly.

IntechOpen
intechopen.com

Built by scientists, for scientists

Explore all IntechOpen books

Meet the editor

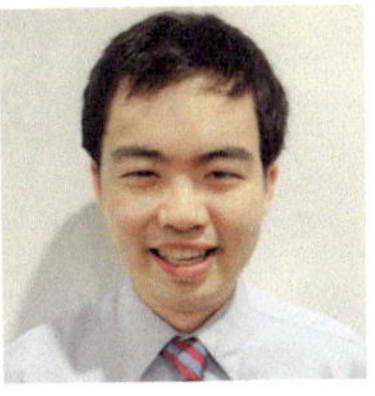

Dr. Henry H. L. Wu, MBChB Ph.D., is a Clinician-Scientist based at Royal North Shore Hospital and the Kolling Institute of Medical Research, The University of Sydney, Australia, and a visiting researcher at the University of New South Wales, Australia. Dr. Wu has published widely in key journals and presented at major international nephrology conferences, and is currently the associate editor of *Nutrition and Health*, review editor of the nephrology section of *Frontiers in Medicine*, and an editorial board member of *BMC Nephrology* and *PloS One*. Dr. Wu is also currently a member of the International Society of Nephrology CardioRenal Toolkit Workgroup. He was elected for full membership to Sigma Xi, The Scientific Honor Research Society, in May 2023.

Contents

Preface

Chronic kidney disease (CKD) is a global health problem with a substantial burden on worldwide health systems and economies, currently affecting more than 10% of the worldwide population. CKD has been projected to become the fifth leading cause of mortality worldwide by 2040. Within the nephrology field, immense efforts and resources have been invested in improving the mechanistic understanding of disease processes, diagnostic approaches, drug therapy options, and personalized treatment strategies related to CKD. The past decade has seen significant breakthroughs in CKD research, namely drugs such as sodium-glucose transport protein two inhibitors and non-steroidal mineralocorticoid antagonists showing promise in slowing disease progression and reducing cardiovascular risks in CKD, and artificial intelligence-driven diagnostics and novel biomarkers enhancing early detection and risk stratification of CKD. Otherwise, there has also been noticeable developments in our scientific community's understanding of pathophysiological processes defining the factors affecting CKD progression; the impact of CKD on nutrition status and vice-versa aka the impact of nutritional deficiencies and supplementation on CKD progression; novel nutritional options to improve the state of the gut-kidney axis; advancing knowledge and management of calcific uremic arteriopathy, often deemed difficult to treat in advanced CKD patients; embracing the existence and clinical significance of the cardio-kidney-metabolic syndrome entity and how to optimize patient care within these contexts; improving hemodialysis access for patients with end-stage kidney disease. This book presents an updated perspective on the various facets of CKD research and clinical practice, featuring chapters written by international authors with expertise in their respective fields.

Dr. Henry H.L. Wu
Royal North Shore Hospital and The University of Sydney,
Sydney, Australia

Chapter 1

From Silent Damage to Inevitable Decline: Unraveling the Progression of CKD

Shimaa Shabaka

Abstract

Chronic kidney disease progression involves a cascade of maladaptive responses to sustained kidney injury, ultimately leading to irreversible nephron loss and end-stage kidney disease (ESKD). Regardless of the initial cause, persistent damage triggers glomerular hypertension, hyperfiltration, and proteinuria, which accelerate further nephron loss. Tubular epithelial cells respond to filtered proteins and ischemia by releasing proinflammatory and pro-fibrotic cytokines (e.g., TGF-β and IL-6), promoting interstitial inflammation and fibrosis. Key markers of progression include declining eGFR and increasing albuminuria. Biomarkers such as KIM-1, Neutrophil gelatinase-associated lipocalin (NGAL), suPAR, and uromodulin offer insights into tubular injury and may improve risk stratification alongside tools like the kidney failure risk equation (KFRE). Management aims to slow progression by addressing hemodynamic and inflammatory pathways. Renin-angiotensin-aldosterone system (RAAS) inhibitors remain foundational. Sodium-glucose cotransporter 2 inhibitors (SGLT2i) have demonstrated renoprotective effects independent of glycemic control. Finerenone, a nonsteroidal mineralocorticoid receptor antagonist, has shown benefit in reducing fibrosis and cardiovascular events. Emerging therapies targeting inflammation, fibrosis, and mitochondrial dysfunction (e.g., bardoxolone and anti-TGF-β agents) are under investigation. Omics-based research is uncovering novel molecular pathways and potential therapeutic targets.

Keywords: CKD, progression, risk factors, biomarkers, management

1. Introduction

Chronic kidney disease (CKD) is a growing public health epidemic with an estimated prevalence of 10.6–13.4%. It is associated with a significant increase in cardiovascular events and mortality [1]. The relentless march of CKD toward end-stage kidney disease (ESKD) places an ever-growing strain on healthcare systems as more patients require costly and complex renal replacement therapies.

CKD progression is driven by a self-perpetuating cycle of nephron loss, where hemodynamic stress and molecular signaling accelerate kidney damage. As the glomerular filtration rate declines, surviving nephrons face increased pressure, triggering hyperfiltration, endothelial injury, and podocyte loss. This cascade stimulates cytokine release, including TGF-β, leading to irreversible replacement of functional kidney tissue with a scar-like extracellular matrix. Despite initial repair attempts, this maladaptive response ultimately seals the fate of the kidney, propelling CKD toward ESKD [2].

Lifestyle modification is a key strategy for slowing CKD progression and reducing associated complications. Guidelines from KDIGO and the American College of Cardiology emphasize the importance of dietary patterns, physical activity, weight management, and avoidance of harmful substances such as tobacco and excessive alcohol [3].

Therapeutic strategies to control CKD progression focus on controlling risk factors, reducing complications, and preserving kidney function. ACEIs/ARBs are cornerstone therapies, effectively lowering blood pressure, reducing proteinuria, and slowing CKD progression while also improving cardiovascular outcomes. Diuretics help manage salt and water retention, alleviating hypertension and volume overload. In recent years, groundbreaking therapies such as SGLT2 inhibitors and nonsteroidal MRAs have emerged, demonstrating significant renal and cardiovascular benefits in large-scale randomized controlled trials. These agents, along with novel endothelin receptor antagonists and GLP-1 receptor agonists, provide additional protective mechanisms beyond traditional RAAS blockade [4].

2. Risk factors for CKD progression

Multiple modifiable and non-modifiable risk factors are associated with CKD progression. Non-modifiable factors include demographic and genetic factors while non-modifiable factors include metabolic, cardiovascular, lifestyle, and other factors.

2.1 Non-modifiable factors

Demographic and genetic factors increase susceptibility and progression of CKD. Studies indicate that individuals residing in low-income regions or areas with limited access to healthcare services have a higher risk of CKD progression. Additionally, racial and ethnic disparities contribute to CKD progression, with African Americans and Hispanics experiencing a greater risk of disease progression compared to Caucasians. This disparity is partially attributed to genetic factors, such as the APOL1 gene, which is more prevalent in African American populations and has been strongly associated with an increased risk of kidney diseases [5]. Genetic predisposition further influences CKD progression through variants such as those in the uromodulin gene [6].

Age is another critical non-modifiable factor, as CKD prevalence increases with advancing age due to cumulative kidney damage and decreased regenerative capacity. Furthermore, sex differences have been observed, with men generally exhibiting a higher risk of CKD progression compared to women, potentially due to hormonal influences and differences in baseline kidney function [7].

Another key non-modifiable determinant is birth weight. Epidemiological studies suggest that low birth weight is associated with an increased risk of CKD in adulthood, possibly due to impaired nephron development and subsequent reduced renal reserve [8].

2.2 Modifiable factors

Lifestyle and behavioral factors, including smoking, diet, physical activity, and substance abuse, play a substantial role in CKD progression. Smoking exacerbates kidney damage by increasing oxidative stress, inducing endothelial dysfunction, and elevating blood pressure. Dietary habits also significantly influence CKD risk, with excessive sodium intake, processed foods, and unhealthy fats contributing to hypertension and metabolic disorders. Conversely, a diet rich in fruits, vegetables, and whole grains has been shown to preserve kidney function. Regular physical activity not only aids in blood pressure regulation but also improves overall cardiovascular and metabolic health, reducing CKD risk.

Cardiovascular disorders, including hypertension, heart failure, and atrial fibrillation, are also significant modifiable risk factors. Hypertension, in particular, has been well-established as a primary contributor to CKD due to its damaging effects on renal vasculature, leading to a progressive decline in kidney function. Blood pressure management is crucial in slowing CKD progression, with some studies suggesting that nocturnal non-dipping blood pressure patterns may serve as an independent risk factor. However, the optimal blood pressure targets for CKD patients remain a subject of debate. Additionally, heart failure and atrial fibrillation contribute to CKD by reducing renal perfusion, exacerbating ischemic kidney injury [9].

Several metabolic factors have been implicated in CKD progression, including fibroblast growth factor 23 (FGF23), serum bicarbonate levels, urinary oxalate, serum uric acid, and parathyroid hormone levels. Elevated FGF23 levels have been associated with increased cardiovascular morbidity and mortality together with accelerated CKD progression, due to their role in phosphate homeostasis and endothelial dysfunction. Similarly, disturbances in acid-base balance, particularly metabolic acidosis, contribute to kidney damage by promoting tubulointerstitial fibrosis. Abnormalities in urinary oxalate and serum uric acid levels can lead to nephrotoxicity and crystal deposition, further accelerating renal decline. Addressing these metabolic imbalances through dietary modifications, pharmacologic interventions, and electrolyte management is a therapeutic target [10, 11].

Several additional factors influence CKD progression, including AKI episodes, degree of renal fibrosis, gut-renal axis, inflammation, and pregnancy. AKI significantly increases the risk of CKD progression through rapid decline of baseline glomerular filtration rate (GFR), associated ischemic and nephrotoxic pathophysiological causes [12]. Renal fibrosis associated with chronic inflammation is a key determinant of CKD progression [13]. The gut-renal axis has emerged as a critical factor in CKD pathophysiology, with dysbiosis contributing to systemic inflammation and uremic toxin production. Modulating gut microbiota through probiotics and dietary strategies may offer therapeutic benefits [13]. Chronic inflammatory states, including autoimmune disorders, further accelerate CKD progression, necessitating targeted immunomodulatory treatments. Additionally, pregnancy poses unique challenges, as CKD increases the risk of complications such as pre-eclampsia and preterm birth, underscoring the need for specialized monitoring and management strategies [14]. Furthermore, puberty has been identified as a period of accelerated glomerular filtration rate (GFR) decline, highlighting the importance of early intervention in at-risk populations [15].

3. Pathophysiology of CKD progression

3.1 Proteinuria as a powerful indicator and prognostic predictor of CKD progression

Proteinuria is a crucial indicator of kidney damage and a significant risk factor for CKD progression. Studies have shown a strong correlation between degree of proteinuria and the rate of kidney function decline [16]. In a large-scale screening of over 107,000 participants in Okinawa, Japan, proteinuria was identified as the most powerful predictor of end-stage kidney disease (ESKD) over a 10-year period [17]. The underlying mechanisms include direct damage to renal tubules, leading to inflammation and fibrosis. Activating the renin-angiotensin-aldosterone system (RAAS) and increased oxidative stress, both of which also accelerate kidney damage [18].

Beyond kidney disease, proteinuria is also associated with a higher risk of cardiovascular complications, including heart failure, myocardial infarction, and stroke. While shared risk factors like hypertension and diabetes play a role, proteinuria itself exacerbates cardiovascular risk through mechanisms such as endothelial dysfunction and increased arterial stiffness [19].

3.2 Visceral obesity and dyslipidemia

Visceral obesity and associated dyslipidemia contribute to renal injury through a complex pathophysiological process primarily involving altered renal hemodynamics and structural changes within the glomerulus. Increased body fat leads to hyperfiltration and glomerulomegaly, causing mechanical stress on podocytes, which are unable to adapt to the expanding glomerular surface. This stress results in podocyte detachment from the glomerular basement membrane, progressing to focal segmental glomerulosclerosis (FSGS). These changes mark the onset of obesity-related glomerulopathy (ORG), which is clinically characterized by proteinuria and declining glomerular filtration rate (GFR) [20]. It also can exert mechanical compression on key renal structures such as the thin loop of Henle and the vasa recta, impairing tubular flow with activation of RAAS leading to disrupted tubulo-glomerular feedback, increased sodium reabsorption and a compensatory rise in renal blood flow, hence GFR [21].

Additionally, excessive accumulation of perirenal fat within the renal sinus exerts direct cytotoxic effects on renal tissue through intracellular buildup of triglycerides and bioactive lipids like ceramides. These toxic metabolites contribute to oxidative stress, trigger the release of proinflammatory cytokines, and are linked to adverse cardiovascular outcomes. Elevated plasma ceramide levels have also been independently associated with CKD progression, irrespective of other comorbidities [22].

3.3 Insulin resistance and uncontrolled blood glucose level

Impaired insulin signaling disrupts the phosphoinositide 3-kinase-protein kinase B (Akt)-endothelial nitric oxide synthase (PI3K-Akt-eNOS) pathway, reducing NO bioavailability and promoting endothelial dysfunction, vasoconstriction, and oxidative stress. Concurrently, antidiuretic effects of insulin resistance increase sodium retention, activate RAAS, and contribute to renal tubular lipid accumulation [23]. This is compounded by the overexpression of tumor growth factor-β1 (TGF-β1) and sterol regulatory element binding protein-1 (SREBP-1), which promote mesangial proliferation, lipid droplet deposition, tubular atrophy, and interstitial fibrosis. Inadequate glycemic control further exacerbates renal injury *via* the formation of advanced glycation end-products (AGEs), which engage RAGE receptors, triggering proinflammatory cascades and oxidative damage [24]. These mechanisms, in conjunction with sympathetic overactivity and impaired baroreflex sensitivity—particularly in obesity-related conditions like obstructive sleep apnea—drive the development of treatment-resistant hypertension and progressive CKD [25].

3.4 Hypertension and chronic inflammation

Hypertension contributes significantly to the onset and progression of CKD through a multifactorial interplay involving neurohormonal activation, sodium retention, and endothelial dysfunction. The overactivity of RAAS, the sympathetic nervous system, and impaired baroreceptor function result in increased systemic and intraglomerular pressure. This promotes glomerular hyperfiltration and mechanical stress on the glomerular capillaries, which ultimately leads to podocyte injury, proteinuria, and glomerulosclerosis. Additionally, aldosterone-induced activation of the mineralocorticoid receptor promotes vasoconstriction, sodium retention, oxidative stress, and pro-fibrotic signaling, all of which contribute to vascular remodeling and renal fibrosis, worsening kidney function over time [26, 27].

Chronic low-grade inflammation, particularly in the setting of obesity and metabolic syndrome, plays a crucial role in the pathogenesis of CKD. Adipose tissue functions as an endocrine organ, releasing adipokines (e.g., leptin and resistin) and proinflammatory cytokines (e.g., TNF-α, IL-6, and MCP-1), which lead to endothelial dysfunction, oxidative stress, and immune cell infiltration in renal tissues. This inflammatory environment promotes the activation of reactive oxygen species (ROS), causing mitochondrial dysfunction, apoptosis of renal tubular cells, and progressive interstitial fibrosis. Furthermore, increased leptin levels stimulate the hypothalamic melanocortin system, enhancing sympathetic activity and contributing to hypertension and renal injury. Together, chronic inflammation and immune dysregulation accelerate structural damage, glomerular sclerosis, and functional decline in CKD [28, 29].

4. Biomarkers predicting CKD progression

4.1 Traditional markers

Several biomarkers have been identified for predicting CKD progression, with traditional markers such as serum creatinine and albuminuria being widely accepted and integrated into the KDIGO classification system. Progressive rising serum creatinine and albuminuria levels are strongly associated with an increased risk of CKD progression. These biomarkers serve as standard clinical tools for assessing kidney function and disease severity.

4.2 Emerging inflammatory and tubular injury biomarkers

Beyond traditional markers, several novel biomarkers have been investigated for their potential role in predicting CKD progression. Tumor necrosis factor receptors 1 and 2 (TNFR1 and TNFR2) are receptors for TNF-α, a proinflammatory cytokine implicated in kidney damage. Elevated levels of these receptors have been linked to increased inflammation and renal function decline, although their independent predictive value has not yet been confirmed in large-scale cohort studies or randomized clinical trials [30]. Similarly, soluble urokinase-type plasminogen activator receptor (suPAR) is a marker of systemic inflammation that has been associated with CKD progression, but it remains unvalidated in multiple independent studies [31].

Several biomarkers specific to tubular injury have also been explored. Kidney injury molecule-1 (KIM-1) is a marker of proximal tubule damage and has been correlated with CKD progression, but its clinical utility as an independent predictor remains uncertain [32]. Neutrophil gelatinase-associated lipocalin (NGAL), another marker of tubular injury initially identified in AKI, has also been detected at elevated levels in CKD patients, yet its independent prognostic value is still under investigation [33].

Liver-type fatty acid-binding protein (L-FABP), a biomarker of oxidative stress and tubular injury, has shown potential in predicting CKD progression but requires further validation [34].

4.3 Other investigational biomarkers

Additional biomarkers with potential relevance to CKD progression include uromodulin (UMOD), a kidney-derived protein involved in renal function and tubular integrity. While UMOD levels have been associated with CKD progression in several studies, their predictive capacity remains unverified in randomized trials [35].

Alpha-1-microglobulin (a1M) has been explored as a marker of tubular injury, showing associations with CKD progression, yet lacking independent validation [36].

MicroRNAs have emerged as promising molecular markers, particularly in diabetic nephropathy, providing insight into gene regulation mechanisms in CKD. Furthermore, the CKD273 panel, a urinary proteomic signature consisting of 273 peptides, has demonstrated strong predictive value for CKD progression, particularly in diabetic nephropathy. Unlike most emerging biomarkers, the CKD273 panel has been validated in multiple cohort studies, making it one of the few widely recognized and clinically applicable biomarkers for CKD progression [37].

5. Prognostic models for CKD progression

Prognostic models play a crucial role in predicting the progression of CKD and guiding clinical decision-making. These models integrate multiple risk factors and biomarkers to estimate the likelihood of adverse renal outcomes.

5.1 Kidney failure risk equation (KFRE)

The KFRE is a widely used prognostic model designed to predict the risk of kidney failure in patients with CKD.

It incorporates key clinical variables, including:

- Age
- Sex
- Estimated glomerular filtration rate (eGFR)
- Urine albumin-to-creatinine ratio (UACR)

More advanced variations of the KFRE include additional laboratory parameters and emerging biomarkers to enhance predictive accuracy [38].

5.2 Chronic kidney disease prognosis consortium (CKD-PC) risk tools

CKD-PC has developed online risk prediction tools for clinical application. These models integrate data from large, diverse cohorts and have been validated in multiple populations. They assess the risk of CKD progression and associated adverse outcomes by considering a broad range of factors, including:

- Traditional risk factors (e.g., eGFR, UACR, and age).
- Comorbid conditions (e.g., hypertension, cardiovascular disease, and diabetes).
- Biomarkers and disease-specific indicators in select patient subgroups [39].

5.3 Advanced ultrasound diagnostic tools for predicting CKD progression

Ultrasound remains the most widely utilized imaging modality in the evaluation of CKD, owing to its non-invasive nature, availability and absence of ionizing radiation. Traditionally, it has been employed to assess kidney macrostructure and to exclude obstructive uropathy. With the advent of high-frequency probes, more detailed visualization of renal parenchyma became possible, while advances in Doppler ultrasound enabled the assessment of segmental arterial flow patterns, including the calculation of resistive indices. These indices serve as indirect markers of microcirculatory impedance, with elevated values associated with progressive renal dysfunction and fibrosis.

More recently, low-flow detection technologies and matrix array probes have enhanced the resolution of parenchymal and microvascular structures. Additionally, contrast-enhanced ultrasound has facilitated the evaluation of renal perfusion. Notably, super-resolution ultrasound imaging, a technique currently undergoing clinical translation, offers unparalleled morphological and functional characterization of renal microcirculation. These technological advancements are further supported by the rapid evolution of radiomics and machine learning, which enhance image acquisition, processing, and the detection and characterization of renal lesions [40].

6. Effective management strategies for slowing CKD progression

CKD requires a multifaceted approach to slow its progression and improve patient outcomes. This includes lifestyle modification, pharmacological treatment, and surgical options in some cases. All these strategies aim to reduce kidney stress, manage comorbidities, and preserve kidney function.

6.1 Lifestyle modification

6.1.1 Dietary interventions

Low-protein diet (LPD) plays a critical role in CKD management by reducing glomerular hyperfiltration and intraglomerular pressure, thereby minimizing kidney damage. It also helps mitigate metabolic acidosis and hyperphosphatemia, which are commonly associated with CKD progression. Furthermore, a plant-dominant LPD has shown potential in modulating the gut microbiome and reducing the production of uremic toxins, further protecting kidney function [41].

Sodium restriction is essential due to its impact on blood pressure regulation and fluid balance. Excessive sodium intake contributes to hypertension, fluid retention, and increased proteinuria, all of which accelerate renal function decline. Reducing dietary sodium has been shown to lower blood pressure and decrease renal workload, ultimately improving kidney health. However, with the introduction of advanced pharmacological therapies, the role of sodium restriction may vary among individuals. Despite this, a balanced diet with controlled sodium intake remains a fundamental strategy in CKD management [42].

Caloric restriction and increased physical activity play a crucial role in preventing and slowing CKD progression in overweight individuals [43].

6.2 Pharmacological treatment

- Renin–angiotensin system inhibitors (RASi), including angiotensin-converting enzyme inhibitors (ACEi) and angiotensin receptor blockers (ARBs), are cornerstone therapies for CKD management. These agents have an integral role in controlling blood pressure, reducing proteinuria, and inhibiting inflammatory cascade modulated by active RAS, thereby slowing CKD progression and improving cardiovascular risk. Optimal therapeutic benefit often requires uptitration to the maximum tolerated dose; however, this is frequently limited by the risk of hyperkalemia. In such cases, rather than reducing or discontinuing RAAS inhibitors, concurrent use of potassium-lowering agents such as sodium zirconium cyclosilicate can be considered. This strategy allows the maintenance of effective RAAS blockade while mitigating the risk of hyperkalemia and preserving renal function [44].

- Sodium-glucose cotransporter-2 inhibitors (SGLT2i), such as dapagliflozin and empagliflozin, have emerged as effective nephroprotective agents. They can reduce glomerular hyperfiltration, lower intraglomerular pressure, and provide direct renal protection beyond their glucose-lowering effects. Clinical trials have shown that SGLT2i significantly slow CKD progression and reduce cardiovascular risk in diabetic and non-diabetic patients. SGLT2i have demonstrated a favorable safety and tolerability profile; however, certain adverse effects must be considered. These include an increased risk of mycotic genital infections, particularly in women, which can be effectively managed through patient education on proper hygiene and early treatment. Although rare, SGLT2i-associated ketoacidosis remains a potential concern, especially in high-risk individuals such as those with insulin deficiency, undergoing surgical stress, experiencing caloric restriction, or engaging in alcohol abuse. Current guidelines recommend temporary discontinuation of SGLT2 inhibitors during periods of heightened risk (e.g., surgery and prolonged fasting) with prompt reinitiation once resolved [45].

- Glucagon-like peptide-1 receptor agonists (GLP-1 RAs), including semaglutide, offer additional kidney protection through their anti-inflammatory and metabolic effects. These agents improve glycemic control, reduce oxidative stress, and lower systemic inflammation. Their role is particularly beneficial in patients with type 2 diabetes and CKD, where metabolic dysregulation exacerbates renal decline [46].

- Selective mineralocorticoid receptor antagonists (MRAs), such as finerenone, have demonstrated significant benefits in reducing albuminuria and inflammation. These agents help prevent fibrotic and inflammatory pathways, thereby slowing CKD progression, particularly in patients with diabetic kidney disease (DKD). So, In patients with type 2 diabetes mellitus, an eGFR >25 mL/min/1.73 m^2, normal serum potassium levels, and persistent albuminuria (>30 mg/g), the addition of a nonsteroidal MRA may provide further renal and cardiovascular protection [47].

- Endothelin-A receptor antagonists (ERAs), such as atrasentan, represent an emerging class of nephroprotective agents targeting renal fibrosis and vascular dysfunction. By inhibiting endothelin-A receptor activity, these drugs reduce proteinuria and inflammation, which are major contributors to CKD progression. Although still under investigation, ERAs hold promise as a future therapeutic option for CKD patients [48].

- Anti-fibrotic agents, including microRNAs, are being explored as novel therapeutic options for CKD. These agents target fibrosis-related pathways, modulating gene expression to reduce renal scarring and inflammation. While still in the experimental phase, anti-fibrotic therapies represent a potential breakthrough in CKD treatment [49].

- Combination therapy involving RAS inhibitors, SGLT2 inhibitors, and MRAs has been suggested as a more effective approach to slowing CKD progression by targeting multiple pathogenic pathways. Clinical trials continue to investigate the benefits of multimodal pharmacological interventions in improving renal outcomes [50].

- Essential amino acids nitrogen-free analogs (EAA-NFAs) have emerged as a strategic adjunct in the dietary management of patients with CKD. These compounds are structurally similar to essential amino acids but lack the nitrogen component, allowing for incorporation into metabolic pathways *via* transamination without increasing the nitrogen burden. The so-called "keto diet" denotes the combination of low-protein diets (0.6 g/kg/day) or very-low-protein diets (VLPDs) (0.3–0.4 g/kg/day) with EAA-NFAs, thereby reducing nitrogen intake while preserving protein synthesis and preventing malnutrition. Clinical evidence suggests that such regimens, when adhered to by well-nourished individuals with low comorbidity burden, can delay CKD progression and reduce the incidence of renal death. Meta-analytical data further support the benefits of EAA-NFA-supplemented diets in delaying the need for dialysis, improving mineral and bone metabolism, and maintaining blood pressure control without adverse effects on nutritional status. A recent meta-analysis comprising 15 clinical trials and a total of 1596 individuals with CKD stages 3–5 assessed the efficacy of VLPDs supplemented with EAA-NFAs in comparison to standard LPDs. Patients receiving EAA-NFA supplementation demonstrated significant improvements in key renal function parameters, including an increase in eGFR and reductions in serum creatinine and BUN levels. Additionally, a significant decrease in PTH concentration was observed, indicating improved mineral metabolism. Notably, no significant changes were reported in serum albumin, cholesterol, phosphorus, or calcium, suggesting that EAA-NFA-supplemented diets are metabolically safe and do not adversely affect nutritional status [51].

6.3 Surgical options

Obesity and CKD progression: Obesity is a well-established risk factor for CKD, contributing to glomerular hyperfiltration, insulin resistance, and systemic inflammation. Excess body weight exacerbates CKD progression by increasing renal workload and metabolic dysfunction. Interventions such as bariatric surgery, particularly sleeve gastrectomy, have been shown to significantly improve renal outcomes in obese patients by promoting weight loss, reducing blood pressure, and enhancing metabolic control.

6.4 Herbal remedies as an adjunctive therapeutic tool for reducing CKD progression

Herbal remedies have shown significant potential in reducing CKD progression through controlling of its key risk factors.

6.4.1 Blood pressure control

Certain plant extracts, such as ergone from *Polyporus umbellatus* and pachymic acid B from *Poria cocos*, have been found to suppress RAS. Additionally, antioxidants and anti-inflammatory properties from natural sources play a role in reducing oxidative stress and vascular damage. Pomegranate juice (*Punica granatum*), for instance, has demonstrated antihypertensive effects in hemodialysis patients by mitigating oxidative damage [52]. Similarly, garlic (*Allium sativum*) has been shown in randomized trials to exert hypotensive effects by enhancing nitric oxide (NO) production, promoting vasodilation, and reducing low-density lipoprotein (LDL) levels, thereby lowering cardiovascular risks [53].

Other plant-based compounds, such as flavonoids in *Theobroma cacao* and nitrate-rich beet (*Beta vulgaris*) juice, have exhibited BP-lowering effects through vasodilation and improving endothelial function. Potential side effects such as gastrointestinal irritation, allergic reactions, and mild digestive discomfort should be considered when using these remedies [54].

6.4.2 Blood glucose reduction in DM

Herbal remedies have a role in lowering blood glucose levels and improving metabolic parameters, which is crucial in preventing DKD. A study comparing Zishentongluo, a traditional herbal decoction, with benazepril in patients with early-stage DKD showed that the herbal treatment significantly improved HbA1C, fasting blood glucose (FBG), total cholesterol, triglycerides (TGs), urine albumin excretion rate (UAER), and renal function markers, outperforming benazepril [55]. Similarly, the Yiqi Huaju Qingli formula, when combined with Western medicine, showed superior effects in reducing body mass index (BMI), waist circumference, insulin resistance, microalbuminuria, and lipid levels, with notable improvements in TG reduction and glycemic control [56].

6.4.3 Lipid profile improvement

Dyslipidemia is a common complication in CKD patients, which contributes to disease progression due to the proatherogenic effect. Some herbal remedies have shown promising effects in improving lipid metabolism and reducing cardiovascular risks. For instance, Xuezhitong capsules, derived from *Allium macrostemon* Bunge, were studied in CKD patients with dyslipidemia and demonstrated a significant reduction in total cholesterol, TGs, and LDL-C while increasing high-density lipoprotein cholesterol (HDL-C), particularly when combined with atorvastatin [57].

6.4.4 Reduction of proteinuria

Astragalus, a well-known traditional herb, significantly reduced proteinuria in CKD patients after a 3-week treatment [58], with a similar effect observed in another study on stage 4 and 5 CKD patients [59]. Furthermore, a combination of *Astragalus* and *Angelica* demonstrated a remarkable decrease in proteinuria in patients with GN, with outcomes comparable to those receiving losartan [60]. Additionally, a randomized trial on *Tangshen granules*, which contain multiple herbal components, showed a significant reduction in 24-hour urinary protein excretion in patients with macroalbuminuria, although its effects on microalbuminuria were not statistically significant [61]. Another large-scale study on *Liuwei dihuang* tablets and *Ginkgo biloba* in DKD patients found that these herbal formulations effectively reduced albuminuria over a 2-year period [62].

6.4.5 Reduction of serum uric acid levels

Hyperuricemia is a contributing factor to CKD progression, and herbal treatments have been explored for their potential role in lowering serum uric acid levels through xanthine oxidase inhibition or enhancing uric acid excretion. *Dioscorea collettii* has been shown to lower serum uric acid by modulating uric acid transporters and inhibiting xanthine oxidase activity [63]. Additionally, curcumin from *Curcuma longa* significantly reduced serum uric acid, lipid levels, and oxidative stress in patients with nonalcoholic fatty liver disease [64]. *Plantago psyllium* seeds, derived from *Plantago ovata*, have also demonstrated efficacy in lowering serum uric acid levels in diabetic and hyperuricemic patients when used as an adjunct to conventional therapies [65].

6.5 Harmful effects of herbal remedies on CKD progression

While many herbal remedies offer therapeutic benefits, some herbs may exacerbate CKD progression by worsening its risk factors. Several herbs, including *Citrus aurantium* (bitter orange), *Glycyrrhiza glabra* (licorice), *Hypericum perforatum* (St. John's wort), and *Ephedra distachya*, have been associated with increased BP. Bitter orange contains adrenergic compounds that elevate heart rate and BP, while licorice induces mineralocorticoid excess, leading to HTN and hypokalemia [66]. Similarly, St. John's wort may trigger hypertensive crises due to its monoamine oxidase inhibitory effects, and *Ephedra* species contain alkaloids that stimulate the sympathetic nervous system, further elevating blood pressure [67].

Some herbal extracts can also negatively impact glucose metabolism, contributing to insulin resistance and poor glycemic control in DKD patients. For example, St. John's wort has been linked to insulin resistance and glucose uptake impairment, and in one case, its consumption led to acute kidney injury requiring hemodialysis. Similarly, certain fruit juices, such as purple grape juice, pink grapefruit juice, and black tea, have been shown to increase xanthine oxidase activity, leading to elevated serum uric acid levels, which can accelerate CKD progression [54].

7. Artificial intelligence and Machine Learning (ML) as a promising tool for CKD prediction and management

Recent advancements in ML have significantly contributed to the evolution of precision medicine in nephrology. The Nephrotic Syndrome Study Network (NEPTUNE) exemplifies this trend, employing multi-dimensional data analysis in observational cohorts to redefine disease classifications [68]. Although this methodology is still in the developmental phase, it holds great potential for improving early diagnosis and risk stratification in renal pathology. ML applications have particularly excelled in biological image analysis, where they are increasingly regarded as reliable diagnostic tools. In nephrology, ML-driven histopathological assessment is emerging as the gold standard for renal disease identification, improving diagnostic accuracy and impacting therapeutic decision-making. Traditional glomerular assessments—such as light microscopy, morphometric analysis, and electron microscopy—remain time-consuming and subjective, thus driving the demand for automated, standardized approaches [69].

Additionally, AI has shown promise in enhancing the estimation of GFR, a key biomarker in CKD management. Beyond imaging, ML algorithms have been applied to predict CKD progression using routine clinical data. Tangri et al. utilized a Cox proportional hazards model based on electronic health records to forecast kidney failure with high accuracy [70]. Building on this, Norouzi et al. developed a neuro-fuzzy system integrating a decade of longitudinal data to predict CKD progression timelines [71]. Similarly, Perott et al. used unsupervised learning methods to effectively anticipate transitions from stage III to IV CKD. Collectively, these innovations highlight the transformative role of AI and ML in renal diagnostics, prognostication, and personalized patient care [72].

8. Conclusion

CKD progression is driven by interrelated mechanisms of glomerular hyperfiltration, inflammation, fibrosis, and tubular injury, regardless of the initial etiology. While traditional therapies such as RAAS blockade remain essential, recent advances including SGLT2 inhibitors, finerenone, and novel biomarkers are transforming management by targeting both hemodynamic and non-hemodynamic pathways. Continued research into molecular mechanisms and precision medicine holds promise for improving individualized care and delaying kidney failure.

Conflict of interest

No conflict of interest.

DOI: http://dx.doi.org/10.5772/intechopen.1011051

Author details

Shimaa Shabaka
Mansoura University Hospital, Mansoura, Egypt

*Address all correspondence to: shimaashabaka@mans.edu.eg

IntechOpen

© 2025 The Author(s). Licensee IntechOpen. This chapter is distributed under the terms of the Creative Commons Attribution License (http://creativecommons.org/licenses/by/4.0), which permits unrestricted use, distribution, and reproduction in any medium, provided the original work is properly cited.

References

[1] Hill NR, Fatoba ST, Oke JL, Hirst JA, O'Callaghan CA, Lasserson DS, et al. Global prevalence of chronic kidney disease–a systematic review and meta-analysis. PLoS One. 2016;**11**(7):e0158765

[2] Shabaka A, Cases-Corona C, Fernandez-Juarez G. Therapeutic insights in chronic kidney disease progression. Frontiers in Medicine. 2021;**8**:645187

[3] Schrauben SJ, Apple BJ, Chang AR. Modifiable lifestyle behaviors and CKD progression: A narrative review. Kidney360. 2022;**3**(4):752-778

[4] Tarun T, Ghanta SN, Ong V, Kore R, Menon L, Kovesdy C, et al. Updates on new therapies for patients with CKD. Kidney International Reports. 2024;**9**(1):16-28

[5] Freedman BI, Limou S, Ma L, Kopp JB. APOL1-associated nephropathy: A key contributor to racial disparities in CKD. American Journal of Kidney Diseases. 2018;**72**(5):S8-S16

[6] Olinger E, Schaeffer C, Kidd K, Elhassan EA, Cheng Y, Dufour I, et al. An intermediate-effect size variant in UMOD confers risk for chronic kidney disease. Proceedings of the National Academy of Sciences of the United States of America. 2022;**119**(33):e2114734119

[7] Ricardo AC, Yang W, Sha D, Appel LJ, Chen J, Krousel-Wood M, et al. Sex-related disparities in CKD progression. Journal of the American Society of Nephrology. 2019;**30**(1):137-146

[8] Eriksson JG, Salonen MK, Kajantie E, Osmond C. Prenatal growth and CKD in older adults: Longitudinal findings from the Helsinki birth cohort study, 1924-1944. American Journal of Kidney Diseases. 2018;**71**(1):20-26

[9] Dasgupta I, Zoccali CJH. Is the KDIGO systolic blood pressure target< 120 mm Hg for chronic kidney disease appropriate in routine clinical practice? Hypertension. 2022;**79**(1):4-11

[10] De Jong MA, Eisenga MF, Van Ballegooijen AJ, Beulens JW, Vervloet MG, Navis G, et al. Fibroblast growth factor 23 and new-onset chronic kidney disease in the general population: The Prevention of Renal and Vascular Endstage Disease (PREVEND) study. Nephrology, Dialysis, Transplantation. 2021;**36**(1):121-128

[11] Atkinson MA, Ng DK, Warady BA, Furth SL, Flynn JT. The CKiD study: Overview and summary of findings related to kidney disease progression. Pediatric Nephrology. 2021;**36**(3):527-538

[12] See EJ, Jayasinghe K, Glassford N, Bailey M, Johnson DW, Polkinghorne KR, et al. Long-term risk of adverse outcomes after acute kidney injury: A systematic review and meta-analysis of cohort studies using consensus definitions of exposure. Kidney International. 2019;**95**(1):160-172

[13] Humphreys BD. Sox9 flips the switch between regeneration and fibrosis. Kidney International. 2024;**106**(5):781-783

[14] Reynolds ML, Oliverio AL, Zee J, Hendren EM, O'Shaughnessy MM, Ayoub I, et al. Pregnancy history and kidney disease progression among women enrolled in cure glomerulonephropathy. Kidney International Reports. 2023;**8**(4):805-817

[15] Ardissino G, Testa S, Daccò V, Paglialonga F, Viganò S, Felice-Civitillo C, et al. Puberty is associated with increased deterioration of renal function in patients with CKD: Data from the ItalKid Project. Archives of Disease in Childhood. 2012;**97**(10):885-888

[16] Maringhini S, Zoccali CJB. Chronic Kidney Disease Progression—A Challenge. A Challenge Biomedicines. 2024;**12**(10):2203

[17] Iseki K, Ikemiya Y, Iseki C, Takishita S. Proteinuria and the risk of developing end-stage renal disease. Kidney International. 2003;**63**(4):1468-1474

[18] Makhammajanov Z, Gaipov A, Myngbay A, Bukasov R, Aljofan M, Kanbay M. Tubular toxicity of proteinuria and the progression of chronic kidney disease. Nephrology, Dialysis, Transplantation. 2024;**39**(4):589-599

[19] Lancet CKDPC. Association of estimated glomerular filtration rate and albuminuria with all-cause and cardiovascular mortality in general population cohorts: A collaborative meta-analysis. The Lancet. 2010;**375**(9731):2073-2081

[20] Goumenos DS, Kawar B, El Nahas M, Conti S, Wagner B, Spyropoulos C, et al. Early histological changes in the kidney of people with morbid obesity. Nephrology, Dialysis, Transplantation. 2009;**24**(12):3732-3738

[21] Zhang X, Lerman LO. The metabolic syndrome and chronic kidney disease. Translational Research. 2017;**183**:14-25

[22] Salvatore SP, Chevalier JM, Kuo SF, Audia PF, Seshan SV, Practice C. Kidney disease in patients with obesity: It is not always obesity-related glomerulopathy alone. Obesity Research & Clinical Practice. 2017;**11**(5):597-606

[23] Ramirez-Jimenez M, Morales-Palomo F, Moreno-Cabañas A, Alvarez-Jimenez L, Ortega JF, Mora-Rodriguez R, et al. Effects of antihypertensive medication and high-intensity interval training in hypertensive metabolic syndrome individuals. Scandinavian Journal of Medicine & Science in Sports. 2021;**31**(7):1411-1419

[24] Li L, Yang J, Li F, Gao F, Zhu L, Hao J. FBXW7 mediates high glucose-induced SREBP-1 expression in renal tubular cells of diabetic nephropathy under PI3K/Akt pathway regulation. Molecular Medicine Reports. 2021;**23**(4):233

[25] Bertolio R, Napoletano F, Mano M, Maurer-Stroh S, Fantuz M, Zannini A, et al. Sterol regulatory element binding protein 1 couples mechanical cues and lipid metabolism. Nature Communications. 2019;**10**(1):1326

[26] Hall JE, do Carmo JM, da Silva AA, Wang Z, Hall ME. Obesity-induced hypertension: Interaction of neurohumoral and renal mechanisms. Circulation Research. 2015;**116**(6):991-1006

[27] Cortinovis M, Perico N, Ruggenenti P, Remuzzi A, Remuzzi G. Glomerular hyperfiltration. Nature Reviews. Nephrology. 2022;**18**(7):435-451

[28] Esmaili S, Hemmati M, Karamian M. Physiological role of adiponectin in different tissues: A review. Archives of Physiology and Biochemistry. 2020;**126**(1):67-73

[29] Markova I, Miklankova D, Hüttl M, Kacer P, Skibova J, Kucera J, et al. The effect of lipotoxicity on renal dysfunction in a nonobese rat model

of metabolic syndrome: A urinary proteomic approach. Journal Diabetes Research. 2019;**2019**(1):8712979

[30] Arthanarisami A, Komaru Y, Katsouridi C, Schumacher J, Verges DK, Ning L, et al. Acute kidney injury-induced circulating TNFR1/2 elevations correlate with persistent kidney injury and progression to fibrosis. Cells. 2023;**12**(18):2214

[31] Abraham AG, Xu Y, Roem JL, Greenberg JH, Weidemann DK, Sabbisetti VS, et al. Variability in CKD Biomarker Studies: Soluble Urokinase Plasminogen Activator Receptor (suPAR) and Kidney Disease Progression in the Chronic Kidney Disease in Children (CKiD) Study. Kidney Medicine. 2021;**3**(5):712-21 e1

[32] Schmidt IM, Srivastava A, Sabbisetti V, McMahon GM, He J, Chen J, et al. Plasma kidney injury molecule 1 in CKD: Findings from the Boston Kidney Biopsy Cohort and CRIC studies. American Journal of Kidney Diseases. 2022;**79**(2):231-243 e1

[33] Marakala V. Neutrophil gelatinase-associated lipocalin (NGAL) in kidney injury–A systematic review. Clinica Chimica Acta. 2022;**536**:135-141

[34] Khatir DS, Bendtsen MD, Birn H, Nørregaard R, Ivarsen P, Jespersen B, et al. Urine liver fatty acid binding protein and chronic kidney disease progression. Scandinavian Journal of Clinical and Laboratory Investigation. 2017;**77**(7):549-554

[35] Thielemans R, Speeckaert R, Delrue C, De Bruyne S, Oyaert M, Speeckaert MMJD. Unveiling the hidden power of uromodulin: A promising potential biomarker for kidney diseases. Diagnostics (Basel). 2023;**13**(19):3077

[36] Garmaa G, Nagy R, Kói T, To UND, Gergő D, Kleiner D, et al. Panel miRNAs are potential diagnostic markers for chronic kidney diseases: A systematic review and meta-analysis. BMC Nephrology. 2024;**25**(1):261

[37] Schunk SJ, Speer T, Petrakis I, Fliser D. Dickkopf 3—a novel biomarker of the 'kidney injury continuum'. Nephrology, Dialysis, Transplantation. 2021;**36**(5):761-767

[38] Ramspek CL, de Jong Y, Dekker FW, van Diepen M. Towards the best kidney failure prediction tool: A systematic review and selection aid. Nephrology, Dialysis, Transplantation. 2020;**35**(9):1527-1538

[39] Ferguson T, Ravani P, Sood MM, Clarke A, Komenda P, Rigatto C, et al. Development and external validation of a machine learning model for progression of CKD. Kidney International Reports. 2022;**7**(8):1772-1781

[40] Fleig S, Magnuska ZA, Koczera P, Salewski J, Djudjaj S, Schmitz G, et al. Advanced ultrasound methods to improve chronic kidney disease diagnosis. Npj Imaging. 2024;**2**(1):22

[41] Sakaguchi Y, Kaimori J-Y, Isaka YJN. Plant-dominant low protein diet: A potential alternative dietary practice for patients with chronic kidney disease. Nutrients. 2023;**15**(4):1002

[42] Valtuille R. Potential novel benefits of sodium restriction in chronic kidney disease. Current Hypertension Reviews. 2021;**17**(1):59-66

[43] Jaramillo-Morales J, Korucu B, Pike MM, Lipworth L, Stewart T, Headley SA, et al. Effects of caloric restriction and aerobic exercise on circulating cell-free mitochondrial DNA

in patients with moderate to severe chronic kidney disease. American Journal of Physiology. Renal Physiology. 2022;**322**(1):F68-F75

[44] Fularski P, Czarnik W, Frankenstein H, Gąsior M, Młynarska E, Rysz J, et al. Unveiling selected influences on chronic kidney disease development and progression. Cells. 2024;**13**(9):751

[45] Mende CW. Chronic kidney disease and SGLT2 inhibitors: A review of the evolving treatment landscape. Advances in Therapy. 2022;**39**(1):148-164

[46] von Scholten BJ, Kreiner FF, Rasmussen S, Rossing P, Idorn T. The potential of GLP-1 receptor agonists in type 2 diabetes and chronic kidney disease: From randomised trials to clinical practice. Therapeutic Advances in Endocrinology and Metabolism. 2022;**13**:20420188221112490

[47] DeFronzo RA, Bakris GL. Modifying chronic kidney disease progression with the mineralocorticoid receptor antagonist finerenone in patients with type 2 diabetes. Diabetes, Obesity & Metabolism. 2022;**24**(7):1197-1205

[48] Martínez-Díaz I, Martos N, Llorens-Cebrià C, Álvarez FJ, Bedard PW, Vergara A, et al. Endothelin receptor antagonists in kidney disease. International Journal of Molecular Sciences. 2023;**24**(4):3427

[49] Gluba-Sagr A, Franczyk B, Rysz-Górzyńska M, Ławiński J, Rysz JJB. The role of miRNA in renal fibrosis leading to chronic kidney disease. Biomedicine. 2023;**11**(9):2358

[50] Sarafidis PJ. Use of ACEi/ARBs, SGLT2 inhibitors and MRAs can help us reach the therapeutic ceiling in CKD. Clinical Kidney Journal. 2024;**17**(2):sfae014

[51] Imam MS, Alrasheedi LST, AlyamiSAH, AljamaanMMA, AlnaimKSK, Alenzi HMA, et al. A meta-analysis examining the impact of consuming nitrogen-free analogs of essential amino acids on the progression of chronic renal disease. Medicina (Kaunas, Lithuania). 2025;**61**(3):423

[52] Shema-Didi L, Sela S, Ore L, Shapiro G, Geron R, Moshe G, et al. One year of pomegranate juice intake decreases oxidative stress, inflammation, and incidence of infections in hemodialysis patients: A randomized placebo-controlled trial. Free Radical Biology & Medicine. 2012;**53**(2):297-304

[53] Asgharpour M, Khavandegar A, Balaei P, Enayati N, Mardi P, Alirezaei A, et al. Efficacy of oral administration of Allium sativum powder "garlic extract" on lipid profile, inflammation, and cardiovascular indices among hemodialysis patients. Evidence-Based Complementary and Alternative Medicine. 2021;**2021**(1):6667453

[54] AlAhmad MM, Al Namer Y, Palaian S, Alomar MJ. A nephrological perspective of herbal remedies on the progression of chronic kidney disease: A systematic review. Journal of Applied Pharmaceutical Science. 2024;**14**(3):011-025

[55] Ma J, Xu L, Dong J, Wei H, Zhi Y, Ma X, et al. Effects of zishentongluo in patients with early-stage diabetic nephropathy. The American Journal of Chinese Medicine. 2013;**41**(02):333-340

[56] Wang T-z, Chen Y, He Y-m, Fu X-d, Wang Y, Xu Y-q, et al. Effects of Chinese herbal medicine Yiqi Huaju Qingli Formula in metabolic syndrome patients with microalbuminuria: A randomized placebo-controlled trial. Journal of Integrative Medicine. 2013;**11**(3):175-183

[57] Feng Y, Liang W, Liang W, Xiao X, Zhang YJ. Effects of Xue Zhi Tong capsules on chronic kidney disease patients with dyslipidemia. Tropical Journal of Pharmaceutical Research. 2022;**21**(1):177-183

[58] Junfeng S, Hanwei Z, Chong Z. Therapeutic efficacy of Astragalus in patients with chronic glomerulonephritis. Acta Universitatis Medicinalis Secondae Shanghai. 2002;**22**(3):245-247

[59] Okuda M, Horikoshi S, Matsumoto M, Tanimoto M, Yasui H, Tomino YJ. Beneficial effect of Astragalus membranaceus on estimated glomerular filtration rate in patients with progressive chronic kidney disease. Hong Kong Journal of Nephrology. 2012;**14**(1):17-23

[60] Peicheng S, Xuejun Y, Liqun HJ. Effect of Astragali and Angelica particle on proteinuria in Chinese patients with primary glomerulonephritis. Journal of Traditional Chinese Medicine. 2016;**36**(3):299-306

[61] Li P, Chen Y, Liu J, Hong J, Deng Y, Yang F, et al. Efficacy and safety of tangshen formula on patients with type 2 diabetic kidney disease: A multicenter double-blinded randomized placebo-controlled trial. PLoS One. 2015;**10**(5):e0126027

[62] Shi R, Wang Y, An X, Ma J, Wu T, Yu X, et al. Efficacy of co-administration of liuwei dihuang pills and ginkgo biloba tablets on albuminuria in type 2 diabetes: A 24-month, multicenter, double-blind, placebo-controlled, randomized clinical trial. Frontiers in Endocrinology. 2019;**10**:100

[63] Guo Y, Lu H, Gan J, Li D, Gao J, Zhang CJT. Efficacy of Chinese herbal medicine Jiangniaosuan formula for treatment of hyperuricemia: Study protocol for a double-blinded non-inferiority randomized controlled clinical trial. Trials. 2022;**23**(1):1-9

[64] Panahi Y, Kianpour P, Mohtashami R, Jafari R, Simental-Mendía LE, Sahebkar AJ. Curcumin lowers serum lipids and uric acid in subjects with nonalcoholic fatty liver disease: A randomized controlled trial. Journal of Cardiovascular Pharmacology. 2016;**68**(3):223-229

[65] Ebadollahi-Natanzi A, Arab-Rahmatipour GJ. Psyllium together with allopurinol can efficiently reduce the increased serum level of uric acid, creatinine and urea: A case report. Iran Journal of Toxicology. 2017;**11**(4):51-56

[66] Murphy SC, Agger S, Rainey PM. Too much of a good thing: A woman with hypertension and hypokalemia. Clinical Chemistry. 2009;**55**(12):2093-2096

[67] Adibelli Z, Karacay I, Demir M, Duran CJ. St. John's Wort (Hypericum perforatum)-related acute kidney injury. Blood Purification. 2022;**51**(6):520-522

[68] Gadegbeku CA, Gipson DS, Holzman LB, Ojo AO, Song PX, Barisoni L, et al. Design of the Nephrotic Syndrome Study Network (NEPTUNE) to evaluate primary glomerular nephropathy by a multidisciplinary approach. Kidney International. 2013;**83**(4):749-756

[69] Delrue C, De Bruyne S, Speeckaert MM. Application of machine learning in chronic kidney disease: Current status and future prospects. Biomedicine. 2024;**12**(3):568

[70] Tangri N, Stevens LA, Griffith J, Tighiouart H, Djurdjev O, Naimark D, et al. A predictive model for progression of chronic kidney disease to kidney failure. Journal of the American Medical Association. 2011;**305**(15):1553-1559

[71] Norouzi J, Yadollahpour A, Mirbagheri SA, Mazdeh MM, Hosseini SA. Predicting renal failure progression in chronic kidney disease using integrated intelligent fuzzy expert system. Computational and Mathematical Methods in Medicine. 2016;**2016**(1):6080814

[72] Perotte A, Ranganath R, Hirsch JS, Blei D, Elhadad N. Risk prediction for chronic kidney disease progression using heterogeneous electronic health record data and time series analysis. Journal of the American Medical Informatics Association. 2015;**22**(4):872-880

Chapter 2

Nutrition in Chronic Renal Failure

George Metry

Abstract

The kidney plays a major role in protein homeostasis as it regulates the amino acids (AAs) pool by synthesis and degradation. In chronic renal failure, the excretion of protein waste products is impaired, leading to the elevation of uremic toxins in the blood and the appearance of uremic symptoms. Increased production of uremic toxins is also aggravated through their production by gut microbiota. The most important toxins are Indoxyl sulfate and p-cresyl sulfate, which are produced by proteolytic bacterial fermentation of aromatic amino acids in the gut. This raises the idea that nutrition is the cornerstone for the management of chronic renal insufficiency by lowering the protein intake, which limits the generation of uremic toxins. This chapter will discuss the different regimes of dietary protein intake in chronic kidney diseases, the roles of IS and p-cresyl sulfate (PCS) on different body organs and the probabilities of therapeutic options.

Keywords: chronic renal failure, protein nutrition, cresyl sulfate, indoxyl sulfate, intestinal microbiota, therapeutic management

1. Introduction

Nutrition is the mainstay for the management of patients with chronic kidney disease (CKD), which depends on the restriction of proteins in the diet. It has long been recognized that high protein intake has a deleterious impact on renal function in CKD patients by increasing glomerular filtration rate (GFR), leading to progressive glomerular sclerosis [1–3], and also increased risk of proteinuria.

For decades, various health benefits have been attributed to protein restriction in patients with CKD, such as favorable metabolic effects, reduction of proteinuria and uremic symptoms and improvement in insulin sensitivity [4, 5]. These results are explained by the potential decrease in uremic toxin concentrations, which improves renal and metabolic parameters and better uremia control [5]. However, this nutritional strategy has several drawbacks, such as poor compliance and a potential risk of energy-wasting [6].

1.1 Groups of uremic toxins

When kidney function deteriorates, many compounds, the so-called uremic retention solutes, accumulate in the circulation and tissues [7, 8]. As a consequence, the progression of kidney dysfunction affects both the quality of life and survival of the patients (CKD). Uremic retention solutes are, conventionally, classified into three groups based on their physicochemical characteristics [9]. The first group is <500 Da and comprises water-soluble, non-protein–binding, low molecular weight compounds, such as urea and creatinine, and these are usually not toxic. The second group is between 500 and 12,000 Da. It comprises medium molecular weight molecules, such as beta 2-microglobulins. They are often inflammatory markers. The third group is >12,000 Da. It contains proteins with binding capacity, such as indoxyl sulfate (IS), p-cresol or p-cresyl sulfate (PCS) and phenols. The third group is usually by the technique of ultra-performance liquid chromatography.

1.2 Effect of kidney on protein metabolism

The kidney takes part in protein metabolism in normal subjects. Tubular cell hypertrophy sometimes occurs in response to physiological or pathological stimuli [10, 11].

Amino acids supply to the kidney occurs through several mechanisms, including (1) arterial blood flow, (2) the luminal tubular cells and (3) filtration of amino acids from the breakdown of low molecular weight proteins through the glomerulus [12]. It is known that the kidney has the functions of both protein synthesis and to a greater extent protein degradation, as detected by leucine kinetics study. An estimate of the amount of protein degraded daily in normal subjects is about 7 g [13–15]. Provided that there is a good supply of proteins reaching the kidney.

In contrast to fat and carbohydrate, protein intake (especially of animal type) significantly influences renal hemodynamics in healthy individuals [16, 17]. Oral proteins or amino acid infusions are accompanied by increased renal blood flow, glomerular filtration rate and tubular cell hypertrophy. Amino acids preferentially metabolized in splanchnic organs have a more pronounced effect than those peripherally metabolized, such as branched-chain amino acids.

Glomerular and tubular hypertrophy leads to hyperfiltration, which is in association with loss of renal autoregulation, and decreased nephron mass contributes significantly to the development of glomerulosclerosis and interstitial fibrosis [18, 19]. These conditions are characterized by irreversible structural changes to the kidney, which ultimately lead to end-stage renal disease.

1.3 Nitrogen homeostasis

Urea inside the body is synthetized in two steps:(1) separation of the amino group from amino acids, followed by (2) its conversion to urea by the liver.

There is an alternative pathway for urea generation, that is, the breakdown of urea by urease enzyme produced by bacteria in the gastrointestinal tract, according to the formula ($NH2\text{-}CO\text{-}NH2 + H_2O \rightarrow 2NH3 + CO_2$). These bacteria include *Proteus mirabilis, Staphylococcus saprophyticus* and *Helicobacter pylori*. Most of the ammonia generated in this way is transported through the portal vein to the liver, where it is synthetized to urea. Urea is ultimately excreted in urine [20].

Ammonia is synthetized by the proximal tubules of the kidney, through deamination of glutamine to form ammonia. Ammonia requires active secretion of H^+ from the tubules to form ammonium. The kidneys play a crucial role in glutamine metabolism and ammonia production. This process is important for regulating acid-base balance and excreting acids and H^+ in urine [20].

In CKD patients, urinary excretion of ammonium declines significantly, accompanied by acid-base imbalance and an increase in the breath ammonia level [21].

1.4 Regimes of dietary protein in CRF

There are two regimes for protein nutrition in CKD patients: a low-protein diet (LPD) and a very low-protein diet (VLPD). Prescribing one of these depends on the individual response of the patient to which type can ameliorate the uremic symptoms.

Young 1987, documented that patients with advanced CKD can maintain a neutral or slightly positive N balance with protein intakes as low as 0.55–0.6 g/kg [22]. The human body responds to a decrease in protein intake with several sequential metabolic changes including a reduction in amino acid oxidation and a decrease in protein degradation which can compensate for decreased protein intake [22].

However, the presence of metabolic acidosis which often occurs in renal patients impairs protein turnover as it adapts to a low protein intake [23]. When acidosis is corrected, the adaptation of protein metabolism to low-protein diets is corrected [24]. Taken together, these studies suggest that under sufficient energy intake and acidosis is corrected, a low-protein diet containing 0.6–0.7 g protein/kg is nutritionally safe in CKD patients.

Some studies were performed to examine if very low protein diet (VLPD) can be tolerated by renal patients. Brunori et al. reported that VLPD supplemented with essential amino acids and keto acids can be safely used in patients with advanced CKD [25]. In addition, some reports indicate that both protein metabolism and N balance adapt successfully in patients who are compliant with supplemented VLPD. Masud et al. [26] observed that when a supplemented VLPD (0.28 g/protein/kg) was administered to CKD patients, their body N balance was maintained neutral.

In another study, Tom et al. [27] evaluated the long-term adaptive response of six CKD patients to VLPD-supplemented diets. They found the rates of N balance at the end of the study did not change from initial values. This is because of long-term suppression of amino acid oxidation and protein degradation when protein intake is reduced.

2. Aromatic and sulfur amino acids metabolism

Metabolism of some amino acids, which have a clinical significance, is described in this section. These include aromatic amino acids (phenylalanine, tyrosine and tryptophane) and sulfurated amino acids (methionine, cysteine and homocysteine).

2.1 Aromatic amino acids

This group has a ring structure with alternating double bonds characteristic, whereas aliphatic amino acids do not contain a ring structure. Aromatic amino acids are necessary for the synthesis of different proteins in the cells.

2.2 Tyrosine metabolism

Phenylalanine (**Figure 1a**) is an essential amino acids, which cannot be synthesized in the body and need an external supply. Tyrosine (**Figure 1b**) is synthesized by adding hydroxyl group to carbon 3 in the phenyl ring through the enzyme phenylalanine hydroxylase. This enzyme is present in the splanchnic organs, that is, the liver and pancreas. However, it is more abundant in the kidney than in the splanchnic area [28].

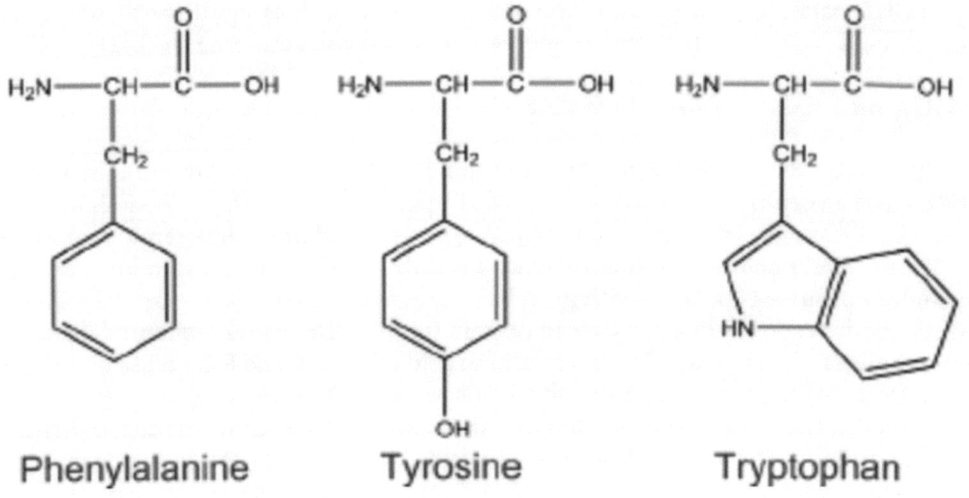

(a) (b) (c)

Figure 1.
Aromatic amino acids which contain a carboxylic acid group (-COOH) attached to an aromatic ring, benzene. They exhibit properties characteristic of both carboxylic acids and aromatic compounds. They include (a) phenylalanine, (b) tyrosine and (c) tryptophane.

Studies indicate that the human kidney plays an important role in the metabolism of tyrosine [29]. Actually, the process of hydroxylation of phenylalanine is greater in the kidney as compared to the splanchnic area [30]. It was found that the whole-body phenylalanine hydroxylation rates are markedly decreased in patients with renal failure. This may explain why tyrosine and the ratio of tyrosine/phenylalanine are almost always reduced in patients with CKD [31]. Production of tyrosine may be also insufficient in some pathological conditions, such as sepsis or liver disease, which are characterized by increased amino acid demand [32].

2.3 Benefits of tyrosine

Tyrosine helps in the synthesis of physiological compounds which contain phenolic group such as dopamine, adrenaline and noradrenaline. Tyrosine is involved in the synthetization of some pituitary hormones.

2.4 Abnormal products of tyrosine

In patients with CKD, tyrosine is transformed to another compound called nitrotyrosine which has deleterious effects on different organs.

2.5 Mechanism of formation of nitrotyrosine

Nitric oxide is produced *in vivo* by the enzyme nitric oxide synthase [32] and probably also by non-enzymic reactions, such as the reaction of nitrites with acid in the stomach. Nitric oxide is used in several metabolic processes in the body. However, it sometimes acts as a cytotoxic or a pathogenetic mediator when there are inflammatory stimuli, one of which is CKD.

NO reacts with superoxide (O2−) from the reactive oxygen species and give peroxynitrite, ONOO−. Peroxynitrate is capable of more nitration of tyrosine to form nitrotyrosine by adding nitro group to C_3 of the phenolic ring. This compound is involved in the pathology of a wide range of diseases, for example, atherosclerosis, rheumatoid arthritis, inflammatory bowel disease, neurodegenerative disease and acute inflammation.

2.6 The kidney and sulfur amino acid metabolism

Methionine is an amino acid containing sulfur residue which is transformed *in vivo* to homocysteine (Hcy), which is further converted to cysteine (Cys). Hcy concentration is usually below 12–15 μM, with higher levels in males [33]. The cysteine concentration level is 240–360 μM.

Cysteine (Cys) is an amino acid which supplies sulfur residue to iron-sulfur proteins. These proteins constitute some important enzymes such as hydrogenase, nitrogenase as well as dehydrogenase/isomerase enzymes. Also, cysteine is required in the formation of pantothenate, which is used to make coenzyme A (CoA), which helps in the metabolism of fatty acids. Cysteine is considered a precursor of glutathione (antioxidation) and taurine which regulate the vital functions of the brain and cardiovascular system.

In the liver, there are two metabolic pathways of cysteine which include (1) the oxidative pathway, which produces at the end pyruvate, or decarboxylation, where the carboxylic group is removed from cysteine and taurine is produced. (2) The desulfated pathway which ends with pyruvate and hydrogen sulfide [34].

2.7 Homocysteine metabolism

Homocysteine (Hcy) is a metabolic intermediate between methionine and cysteine. Physiologically, there is no role of Hcy except as a metabolic product leading to cysteine. However, its elevation in plasma has a toxic effect.

2.7.1 Causes of elevation of homocysteine

It may occur with certain habits like smoking, alcohol, lack of exercise, excess caffeine and old age [35, 36]. High levels of homocysteine are seen in patients with kidney chronic kidney diseases, hypothyroidism, and psoriasis and with certain medications (such as antiepileptic drugs and methotrexate).

The elevated level of Hcy in the body can cause various diseases like decreased renal function [37], ischemic heart disease, ischemic stroke, cerebrovascular and psychiatric diseases like Alzheimer's and autism. The major cause behind these diseases is the increased production of reactive oxygen species, which may cause lipid peroxidation and cell membrane injury [38].

Vitamin B12, vitamin B6 and folate can greatly help decrease the concentration of Hcy in plasma. An inverse relationship has been reported between the concentration of Hcy and these factors in the human body [39]. These elements are present in fruits and vegetables or by medical supplementation.

3. The relationship between the kidney and gut microbiota

There is a reciprocal relationship observed between gut microbiota and chronic kidney disease (CKD), which means that the existence of pathogenic bacteria in the gut leads to progression of renal failure. This is recognized as the "gut-kidney axis" [40].

In humans, the gut microbiota plays an important role in health and diseases [41, 42]. Alterations of the intestinal microbiota, which is termed dysbiosis, are linked to the development of different health problems, such as inflammatory bowel disease, cancer, obesity, diabetes, cardiovascular and kidney disease [43–45]. In normal subjects, gut microbiota acts as a barrier against invading pathogens and augment the immune system. These bacteria have various metabolic functions, such as the fermentation of non-digestible dietary compounds in the large intestine [46, 47].

3.1 Normal physiology of gut microbiota

Several hundreds of bacterial species are inhabitants of the human gut, making up bacterial flora. 99% of these bacteria are anaerobes and obtain their energy through the fermentation of organic compounds, making them more simple products. Anaerobic bacteria are considered normal commensals in the gut. However, under certain conditions, when the host defense becomes weak, anaerobe bacteria become opportunistic pathogens, causing serious infections in any part of the body, especially when they escape their original environment.

Approximately 6–18 grams of proteins enter the large intestine every day, mostly from protein intake in the diet and to a lesser extent from other endogenous sources. The gut bacteria secrete the protease enzyme which causes breakdown of proteins into peptidases, then into small oligopeptides, and further into amino acids. These amino acids are available for assimilation by colon microbiota or can be further metabolized by host enzymes [48].

In the distal part of the colon, the aromatic amino acids phenylalanine, tyrosine and tryptophane are metabolized by bacteria into phenolic compounds, including p-cresyl- and indoxyl sulfate. On entering the circulation, these solutes bind to plasma albumin in a reversible manner and establish a rapid equilibrium between the free and the bound fractions [49]. The solutes are excreted from the kidney, the free fractions are filtered at the glomerulus and the bound fraction is secreted at the site of the tubular epithelial cells, and finally excreted are excreted in urine. In CKD patients, excretion of these solutes is impaired, resulting in their accumulation in the blood.

Chronic kidney disease is almost associated with pathological alterations in gut microbiome composition (gut dysbiosis). This in turn leads to the production of various toxins and metabolites that contribute to uremic toxicity. Toxicity is exacerbated by other factors, such as the gut wall edema, intestinal barrier impairment, translocation of bacteria and endotoxins across the intestinal wall with a resultant systemic inflammation. Two key toxins produced by proteolytic bacterial fermentation in the gut are indoxyl sulfate (IS) and p-cresyl sulfate (PCS) [49].

3.2 Formation of indoxyl- and p-cresyl sulfate

Indoxyl sulfate is a product of tryptophan (**Figure 1c**) metabolism facilitated by Escherichia coli and *Clostridium sporogenes*, while p-Cresyl sulfate is generated by breakdown of tyrosine and phenylalanine by intestinal anaerobes, such as *Clostridium difficile*, *Fecal bacterium prausnitzii*, *Subdoligranulum* and selected strains within the *Bifidobacterium* and *Lactobacillus* genus [49].

The elevated serum levels of indoxyl sulfate and p-cresyl sulfate are conversely associated with CKD progression [50]. The levels of IS may be more than 50 times and PCS more than 15 times compared to that in healthy subjects. Elevations start at the early stage of decreased renal function and become progressively more elevated with advancing severity. These increases in serum levels are associated with adverse renal, metabolic and cardiovascular effects.

3.3 Renal effects

Elevation of serum IS and PCS levels in patients with CKD are associated with CKD progression [51]. The mechanisms underlying the adverse renal effects are thought to be at least partly mediated by the production of reactive oxygen species (ROS), which in turn activate a certain protein called the nuclear factor kappa B pathway (NFκB) [52].

Nuclear factor κB (NF-κB) is a family of proteins which play an important role in different aspects of immune responses. It is vital for normal immune responses against infections. However, deregulated NF-κB activation is a major cause of inflammatory diseases, involving different types of renal injury, infection and autoimmunity.

IS and PCS have also been shown to activate the renin-angiotensin aldosterone cascade. Overactivity of this system results in the rising of glomerular capillary pressure, leading to endothelium vascular injury of the glomerulus which may end with fibrosis [53].

3.4 Metabolic effects

It has been shown that in mouse models, the administration of PCS for 4 weeks has been observed to induce hyperglycemia due to insulin resistance, hypercholesterolemia and fat redistribution to muscle and liver, similar to the metabolic derangements observed in CKD [54].

These metabolic effects appeared to be ameliorated by therapies which reduce uremic toxins, such as the use of the prebiotic agent or low-protein diet. Reduction of serum PCS concentration leads to improved glucose tolerance, insulin resistance, dyslipidemia and ectopic fat distribution in uremic mice [55].

3.5 Cardiovascular effects

Indoxyl sulfate and p-cresyl sulfate cause proliferation of the vascular smooth muscle cells which proceed to atherosclerosis. Spiral computed tomography has revealed aortic calcification in some renal patients with high levels of IS and PCS [56]. Therefore, elevations of these toxins are considered to be predictors of cardiovascular morbidity and mortality.

Observational studies were performed by Lin and colleagues on 1572 patients with stages of 1–5 CKD and followed up to 5 years. The authors found that mortality was significantly associated with the elevation of serum levels of both toxins, although the results were limited by the heterogenicity [57].

3.6 Therapeutic options for reducing IS and PCS in the body

These options are suggested to target the elevated levels of both IS and PCS, which are toxic to both the nephron and vascular system. Potential therapeutic strategies may involve (1) reducing the formation in the gut, (2) inhibiting toxins to traverse the intestinal barriers and (3) increasing excretion by the proximal tubules.

3.7 Reduced gut synthesis

Production of uremic toxins is usually augmented by a high-protein diet and generated through the metabolism of the gut microbiota. Therefore, the prescription of low-protein or very low-protein diet regimens has experienced an interest. The type of regimen is determined by the patient's response.

Marzocco and colleagues investigated a low-protein diet (LPD; 0.6 g/kg/day) versus a very low-protein diet (VLPD; 0.3 g/kg/day) in 32 patients with a creatinine clearance between 20 and 55 ml/min. The authors found that patients treated with a VLPD experienced a significant 36% reduction in serum IS levels compared with those treated with LPD. However, the risks of malnutrition may be present [58]. Also, poor compliance of the participants is likely to be a problem.

3.8 Prebiotics and probiotics

Prebiotic foods contain non-digestible fibers that microorganisms in the gut can break down to obtain energy. Prebiotics are usually present in vegetables, such as whole grains, greens, onions, garlic, soybeans, artichokes and also bananas.

Probiotics are live microorganisms which improve the gut microbiota. Probiotics are thought to help restore the natural balance of bacteria in the gut, especially after being disrupted by illnesses, and also help to overcome the harmful bacteria. Probiotics are mostly lactic acid bacteria, which have been shown to decrease both serum IS concentration by 30% and urinary PCS. Lactic acid bacteria combat the overgrowth and effect of aerobic bacteria.

3.9 Effect of synbiotics on gut bacteria

Synbiotics always represent a combination of both pre- and probiotics [59]. Synbiotic has an effect on the gut microbiome [60], with a significantly increased abundance of: (1) *Bifidobacterium species*. (3.2%), which are gram-positive anaerobic bacteria. These bacteria are one of the major species that make up the gut microbiota, (2) Lachnospiraceae bacteria (2.1%), they are anaerobic, spore-forming bacteria which ferment polysaccharides to fatty acids. These bacteria may protect against colon cancer.

Synbiotics decrease the abundance of Ruminococcaceae (−4.3%), which are gram-positive, anaerobic and related to clostridia. Their abundance is associated with some diseases like inflammatory bowel syndrome and Parkinsons disease.

3.10 Gastrointestinal sequestration

AST-120 (kremezin), is an intestinal adsorbent that binds uremic toxins and their precursors, leading them to be excreted in feces.

3.11 The mechanism of its action

Acarbose is an inhibitor of α-glucosidase enzymes in the intestinal brush border. This maintains polysaccharides in the intestine undigested and blocks their transformation to glucose. In this way, the microbiota activity is shifted to saccharolytic fermentation rather than proteolytic fermentation, with a resulting decrease in uremic toxins.

Evenepoel *et al.* demonstrated that treatment with oral acarbose 300 mg per day for 3 weeks resulted in significant reductions in both serum p-cresol concentration and urinary excretion [61]. However, its side effects of intestinal flatulence limit its use.

3.12 NiaoDuQing granules

NiaoDuQing (NDQ) is a Chinese medicine in the form of granules. This product comprises 10 medicinal herbs and has good pharmacological effects in CKD, which include improving blood chemistry, relieving clinical symptoms and ameliorating renal anemia [62]. It may also prolong the kidney function.

NDQ achieves therapeutic effects through multiple physiological pathways through the effect of the herbal substances. However, the pharmacological mechanisms require more investigation.

3.13 Reduced proximal tubular retention: In the basolateral membrane of the proximal tubu

The kidney has an important role in maintaining blood homeostasis. There are special proteins termed organic anion transporter (OAT), including OAT1 and OAT3. These proteins are present in the basolateral membrane of the cells of the proximal tubules. The proteins play an important part in selective uptake of metabolites and toxins from plasma to the cytoplasm of the proximal tubular cells, then transported to the lumen to be excreted in urine.

Deguchi et al. demonstrated that p-aminohippurate (OAT1 inhibitor), pravastatin (OAT3 inhibitor) and benzylpenicillin (OAT3 inhibitor) could inhibit the renal tubular uptake of indoxyl sulfate and augment its urinary excretion [63].

3.14 Plant proteins

There are strong associations between animal proteins and the progression of renal disease. Animal proteins are often accompanied by increased insulin resistance, microalbuminuria, proteinuria and progression of renal disease. Also, animal diets contain saturated fatty acids which enhance atherosclerosis.

On the other hand, plant diet has several advantages, including a higher intake of fibers, better digestion and good weight control. Plant diet supplies high amount of mono- and polyunsaturated fatty acids, which improve lipid profile.

Phosphorus intake in animal diets differs from that in plant diets. Phosphorus in animal proteins is forming organic phosphates, which are easily hydrolyzed and quickly absorbed from the intestine. Phosphorus of plant origin is mostly in the form of phytic acid or phytate. Therefore, the bioavailability of phosphorus from plant food is fairly low [64, 65].

However, there is a debate that proteins of plant origin would be less sufficient to meet daily protein targets in renal patients, but a number of studies confirmed that it is possible to achieve a target of 1–1.2 g protein/kg/day is recommended in pre uremic patients with a vegetarian diet [66].

3.15 Bone disorder

Adequate calcium, protein and vitamin D are necessary to maintain normal bone density. It appears that the absorption of plant calcium is less efficient due to high phytic and oxalic acids in the plant diet [67].

In addition, there is a lack of vitamin D activation in patients with renal failure. Vitamin D (Cholecalciferol) is taken by diet in the inactive form. In the liver, the OH^- group is added to C_{25} by the enzyme 25-hydroxylase to form

25-hydroxycholecalciferol. In the kidney, another OH^- group is added to C_1 by the enzyme 1-alpha-hydroxylase to form the biologically active vitamin D, 1,25-dihydroxycholecalciferol. The process of renal hydroxylation is deficient in renal failure, leading to osteoporosis. Therefore, supplements of active vitamin D should be taken by renal patients.

3.16 Laxatives

There is a high frequency of constipation in patients with renal failure due to dietary restrictions, sedentary lifestyle and low fluid intake.

In CKD patients, the colonic transit time is prolonged mainly in the ascending colon and in the recto-sigmoid segment [68]. Colonic transit time (CTT) is the time required for feces to pass through the colon. This is measured by X-ray, which traces capsules containing X-ray markers. This test is a basic tool in the diagnosis of patients with constipation. The average normal transit time is 35 hours. The upper limit of normal is 72 hours. If CTT exceeds the upper limit, it indicates colonic inertia.

Longer colonic transit time results in elevated bacterial fermentation of amino acids and, subsequently, an overgrowth of proteolytic bacteria in the human colon. In a study by Roager et al. [68], urinary p-cresyl sulfate is correlated positively with colonic transit time [69]. This means that constipation creates an environment for more bacteria multiplication and, subsequently, more production of p-cresyl sulfate. This raises the possibility that the administration of laxatives, for example, lactulose or macrogol might decrease p-cresyl- and indoxyl sulfate levels in the body.

3.17 Future outlook

Since Indoxyl sulfate and p-cresyl sulfate are potentially uremic toxins which aggravate progression of renal failure, their measurements should be added to the routine nephrological follow-up measurements. They are measured in serum by ultra-performance liquid chromatography, and our recommendation is to be every 3 months.

If serum cresyl and indoxyl sulfate are elevated, this should alarm the doctor that the decreased renal function will proceed to end-stage kidney failure. Accordingly, one or combined regimens should be adopted for lowering these products, including reduced intestinal bacterial production through synbiotics use. Also, laxatives are used to minimize these toxins inside the gut. The patient is advised to minimize proteins and depend mainly on plant proteins. A low-protein diet or very low-protein diet is prescribed when creatinine clearance is around 20 ml/min.

Moreover, we aim to minimize the contents of aromatic amino acids in the protein supply to uremic patients. This can be done through:

1. Modified protein supply in the tablets or liquid form in which aromatic amino acids content can be reduced to 50%.

2. Manufacturing of modified nutrition products which can be sold freely. They contain modified formula of amino acids specifically for renal patients, for example, as dairy products.

DOI: http://dx.doi.org/10.5772/intechopen.1011289

Author details

George Metry[1,2,3,4]

1 Zagazig University, Egypt

2 Science in Internal Medicine, Cairo University, Egypt

3 Internal Medicine, Uppsala University, Sweden

4 Renal Research Institute, New York, USA

*Address all correspondence to: gmetry@hotmail.com

IntechOpen

© 2025 The Author(s). Licensee IntechOpen. This chapter is distributed under the terms of the Creative Commons Attribution License (http://creativecommons.org/licenses/by/4.0), which permits unrestricted use, distribution, and reproduction in any medium, provided the original work is properly cited.

References

[1] Kalantar-Zadeh K, Fouque D. Nutritional management of chronic kidney disease. The New England Journal of Medicine. 2017;**377**:1765-1776

[2] De Miguel C, Lund H, Mattson DL. High dietary protein exacerbates hypertension and renal damage in Dahl SS rats by increasing infiltrating immune cells in the kidney. Hypertension. 2011;**57**:269-274

[3] Jia Y et al. Long-term high intake of whole proteins results in renal damage in pigs. The Journal of Nutrition. 2010;**140**:1646-1652

[4] Hahn D, Hodson EM, Fouque D. Low protein diets for non-diabetic adults with chronic kidney disease. Cochrane Database of Systematic Reviews. 2018;**10**:1-73

[5] Ko GJ, Obi Y, Tortorici AR, Kalantar-Zadeh K. Dietary protein intake and chronic kidney disease. Current Opinion in Clinical Nutrition and Metabolic Care. 2017;**20**:77-85

[6] Noce A et al. Is low-protein diet a possible risk factor of malnutrition in chronic kidney disease patients? Cell Death Discovery. 2016;**2**:16026

[7] Duranton F, Cohen G, de Smet R, Rodriguez M, Jankowski J, Vanholder R, et al. Normal and pathologic concentrations of uremic toxins. Journal of the American Society of Nephrology. 2012;**23**:1258-1270

[8] Vanholder R, de Smet R, Glorieux G, Argiles A, Baurmeister U, Brunet P, et al. Review on uremic toxins: Classification, concentration, and interindividual variability. Kidney International. 2003;**63**:1934-1943

[9] Meyer TW, Hostetter TH. Uremia. The New England Journal of Medicine. 2007;**357**:1316-1325

[10] Vanholder R, Baurmeister U, Brunet P, Cohen G, Glorieux G, Jankowski J. A bench to bedside view of uremic toxins. Journal of the American Society of Nephrology. 2008;**19**:863-870

[11] Garibotto G, Tessari P, Sacco P, Deferrari G. Amino acid metabolism, substrate availability and the control of protein dynamics in the human kidney. Journal of Nephrology. 1999;**12**:203-211

[12] Tessari P, Garibotto G, Inchiostro S, Robaudo C, Saffioti S, Vettore M, et al. Kidney, splanchnic, and leg protein turnover in humans. Insight from leucine and phenylalanine kinetics. The Journal of Clinical Investigation. 1996;**98**:148-192

[13] Garibotto G, Sofia A, Saffioti S, Bonanni A, Mannucci I, Verzola D. Amino acid and protein metabolism in the human kidney and in patients with chronic kidney disease. Clinical Nutrition. 2010;**29**:424-433

[14] Garibotto G, Pastorino N, Dertenois L. Nutritional management of renal diseases. In: Kopple JD, Massry S, editors. Protein and Amino Acid Metabolism in Renal Disease and in Renal Failure. USA: William and Wilkins; 2003. pp. 20-32

[15] Friedman AN. High-protein diets: Potential effects on the kidney in renal health and disease. American Journal of Kidney Diseases. 2004;**44**:950-962

[16] Goldberg A, Guggenheim K. The digestive release of amino acids and their concentrations in the portal

plasma of rats after protein feeding. The Biochemical Journal. 1962;**83**:129-135

[17] Claris-Appiani A, Assael BM, Tirelli AS, Marra G, Cavanna G. Lack of glomerular hemodynamic stimulation after infusion of branched-chain amino acids. Kidney International. 1988;**33**:91-94

[18] Zeisberg M, Strutz F, Müller GA. Renal fibrosis: An update. Current Opinion in Nephrology and Hypertension. 2001;**10**:315320

[19] Hill GS. Hypertensive nephrosclerosis. Current Opinion in Nephrology and Hypertension. 2008;**17**:266270

[20] Bergen WG, Wu G. Intestinal nitrogen recycling and utilization in health and disease. The Journal of Nutrition. 2009;**139**:821-825

[21] Vallet M, Metzger M, Haymann JP, Flamant M, Gauci C, Thervet E, et al. Urinary ammonia and long-term outcomes in chronic kidney disease. Kidney International. 2015;**88**:137-145

[22] Young VR. Kinetics of human amino acid metabolism: Nutritional implications and some lessons. McCollum award lecture. The American Journal of Clinical Nutrition. 1987;**46**:709-725

[23] Williams B, Hattersley J, Layward E, Walls J. Metabolic acidosis and skeletal muscle adaptation to low protein diets in chronic uremia. Kidney International. 1991;**40**:779-786

[24] Bernhard J, Beaufrere B, Laville M, Fouque D. Adaptive response to a low protein diet in predialysis chronic renal failure patients. Journal of the American Society of Nephrology. 2001;**12**:1249-1254

[25] Brunori G, Viola BF, Parrinello G, De Biase V, Como G, Franco V, et al. Efficacy and safety of a very-low-protein diet when postponing dialysis in the elderly: A prospective randomized multicenter controlled study. American Journal of Kidney Diseases. 2007;**49**:569-580

[26] Masud T, Young VR, Chapman T, Maroni BJ. Adaptive responses to very low protein diets: The first comparison of ketoacids to essential amino-acids. Kidney International. 1994;**45**:1182-1199

[27] Tom K, Young VR, Chapman T, Masud T, Apkele L, Maroni BJ. Long-term adaptive responses to dietary protein restriction in chronic renal failure. American Journal of Physiology. Endocrinology and Metabolism. 1995;**268**:E668-E677

[28] Tessari P, Deferrari G, Robaudo C, Vettore M, Pastorino N, De Biasi L, et al. Phenylalanine hydroxylation across the kidney in humans. Kidney International. 1999;**56**:2168-2172

[29] Moller N, Meek S, Bigelow M, Andrews J, Nair KS. The kidney is an important site for in vivo phenylalanine-to-tyrosine conversion in adult humans: A metabolic role of the kidney. Proceedings of the National Academy of Sciences of the United States of America. 2000;**97**:1242-1246

[30] Boirie Y, Albright R, Bigelow M, Nair KS. Impairment of phenylalanine conversion to tyrosine in end-stage renal disease causing tyrosine deficiency. Kidney International. 2004;**66**:591-596

[31] Kopple JD. Phenylalanine and tyrosine metabolism in chronic kidney failure. The Journal of Nutrition. 2007;**137**:1586S-1590S

[32] Lizasoain I, Moro MA, Knowles RG, Darley-Usmar V, Moncada S. Nitric oxide

and peroxynitrite exert distinct effects on mitochondrial respiration which are differentially blocked by glutathione or glucose. The Biochemical Journal. 1996;**314**:877-880

[33] Rehman T, Shabbir M, Inam-Ur-Raheem M, Manzoor MF, Ahmad N, Ahmad H, et al. Cysteine and homocysteine as biomarker of various diseases. Food Science & Nutrition. 2020;**8**:4696-4707

[34] Stipanuk M, Ueki I. Dealing with methionine/homocysteine sulfur. Cystene metabolism to taurine and inorganic sulfur. Journal of Inherited Metabolic Disease. 2011;**34**:17-32

[35] Barroso M, Kao D, Tavares de Almeida I, Castro R, Loscalzo J, Handy DE. S-adenosylhomocysteine induces inflammation through NFkB: A possible role for EZH2 in endothelial cell activation. Biochimica et Biophysica Acta. 2016;**1862**:82-92

[36] Cohen E, Margalit I, Shochat T, Goldberg E, Krause I. Gender differences in homocysteine concentrations, a population-based cross-sectional study. Nutrition, Metabolism and Cardiovascular Diseases. 2019;**29**:9-14

[37] Ganguly P, Alam S. Role of homocysteine in the development of cardiovascular disease. Nutrition Journal. 2015;**10**:14-16

[38] Lehotský J, Tothová B, Kovalská M, Dobrota D, Beňová A, Kalenská D, et al. Role of homocysteine in the ischemic stroke and development of ischemic tolerance. Frontiers in Neuroscience. 2016;**10**:538-553

[39] Ntaios G. Homocysteine, B vitamins, and cardiovascular risk. In: Ross R, editor. Foods and Dietary Supplements in the Prevention and Treatment of Disease in Older Adults. 1st ed. Amsterdam, Netherland: Elsevier/Academic Press; 2015. pp. 309-318

[40] Meijers BK, Evenepoel P. The gut-kidney axis: Indoxyl sulfate, p-cresyl sulfate and CKD progression. Nephrology Dialysis Transplantation. 2011;**26**:759-761

[41] Yao CK, Muir JG, Gibson PR. Review article: Insights into colonic protein fermentation, its modulation and potential health implications. Alimentary Pharmacology & Therapeutics. 2016;**43**:181-196

[42] Gibson SA, McFarlan C, Hay S, MacFarlane GT. Significance of microflora in proteolysis in the colon. Applied and Environmental Microbiology. 1989;**55**:679-683

[43] Smith EA, Macfarlane GT. Dissimilatory amino acid metabolism in human colonic bacteria. Anaerobe. 1997;**3**:327-337

[44] Schepers E, Glorieux G, Vanholder R. The gut: The forgotten organ in uremia? Blood Purification. 2010;**29**:130-136

[45] Meyer TW, Hostetter TH. Uremic solutes from colon microbes. Kidney International. 2012;**81**:949-954

[46] Mafra D, Barros AF, Fouque D. Dietary protein metabolism by gut microbiota and its con sequences for chronic kidney disease patients. Future Microbiology. 2013;**8**:1317-1323

[47] Evenepoel P, Meijers BK, Bammens BR, Verbeke K. Uremic toxins originating from colonic microbial metabolism. Kidney International Supplements. 2009;**76**:S12-S19

[48] Briskey D, Tucker P, Johnson DW, Coombes JS. The role of the gastrointestinal tract and microbiota on uremic toxins and chronic kidney disease development. Clinical and Experimental Nephrology. 2017;**21**(1):7-15

[49] Rossi M, Campbell K, Johnson D, Stanton T, Pascoe E, Hawley C, et al. Uraemic toxins and cardiovascular disease across the chronic kidney disease spectrum: An observational study. Nutrition, Metabolism & Cardiovascular Diseases. 2014;**24**:1035-1042

[50] Koppe L, Pillon NJ, Vella RE, Croze ML, Pelletier CC, Chambert S, et al. p-Cresyl sulfate promotes insulin resistance associated with CKD. Journal of the American Society of Nephrology. 2013;**24**:88-99

[51] Yamamoto H, Tsuruoka S, Ioka T, Ando H, Ito C, Akimoto T, et al. Indoxyl sulfate stimulates proliferation of rat vascular smooth muscle cells. Kidney International. 2006;**69**(10):1780-1785

[52] Zhang H, Sun S-C. Nuclear factor kappa B in inflammation and renal diseases. Cell & Bioscience. 2015;**16**:5-63

[53] Liabeuf S, Barreto DV, Barreto FC, Meert N, Glorieux G, Schepers E, et al. Free p-cresylsulphate is a predictor of mortality in patients at different stages of chronic kidney disease. Nephrology Dialysis Transplantation. 2010;**25**:1183-1191

[54] Sun CY, Chang SC, Wu MS. Uremic toxins induce kidney fibrosis by activating intrarenal renin-angiotensin-aldosterone system associated epithelial-to-mesenchymal transition. PLoS One. 2012;7:1-10

[55] Fouque D, Laville M. Low protein diets for chronic kidney disease in nondiabetic adults. Cochrane Database of Systematic Reviews. 2009;(3):1-26

[56] Lin CJ, Wu V, Wu PC, Wu CJ. Meta-analysis of the associations of p-cresyl sulfate (PCS) and indoxyl sulfate (IS) with cardiovascular events and all-cause mortality in patients with chronic renal failure. PLoS One. 2015;**10**(7):e0132589

[57] Marzocco S, Dal Piaz F, Di Micco L, Torraca S, Sirico ML, Tartaglia D, et al. Very low protein diet reduces indoxyl sulfate levels in chronic kidney disease. Blood Purification. 2013;**35**:196-201

[58] Ikizler TA. Dietary protein restriction in CKD: The debate continues. American Journal of Kidney Diseases. 2009;**53**:189-191

[59] Guida B, Germano R, Trio R, Russo D, Memoli B, Grumetto L, et al. Effect of short-term synbiotic treatment on plasma p-cresol levels in patients with chronic renal failure: A randomized clinical trial. Nutrition, Metabolism & Cardiovascular Diseases. 2014;**24**:1043-1049

[60] Chen L, Shi J, Ma X, Shi D, Qu H. Effects of microbiota-driven therapy on circulating indoxyl sulfate and P-cresyl sulfate in patients with chronic kidney disease: A systematic review and meta-analysis of randomized controlled trials. Advances in Nutrition. 2021;**14**:1267-1278

[61] Evenepoel P, Bammens B, Verbeke K, Vanrenterghem Y. Acarbose treatment lowers generation and serum concentrations of the protein-bound solute p-cresol: A pilot study. Kidney International. 2006;**70**:192-198

[62] Wang X, Suyun Y, Jia Q, Chen L, Zhong J, Pan Y, et al. NiaoDuQing granules relieve chronic kidney disease symptoms by decreasing renal fibrosis and anemia. Oncotarget. 2017;**8**:55920-55937

[63] Deguchi T, Kusuhara H, Takadate A, Endou H, Otagiri M, Sugiyama Y.

Characterization of uremic toxin transport by organic anion transporters in the kidney. Kidney International. 2004;**65**:162-174

[64] Kaimori J-Y, Oka TF, Isaka Y. Plant-dominant low-protein diets: A promising dietary strategy for mitigating disease progression in people with chronic kidney disease. Nutrients. 2025;**4**:643-657

[65] Ferdowsian HR, Barnard ND. Effects of plant-based diets on plasma lipids. The American Journal of Cardiology. 2009;**104**:947-956

[66] Chauveau P, Combe C, Fouque D, Aparicio M. Vegetarianism: Advantages and drawbacks in patients with chronic kidney diseases. Journal of Renal Nutrition. 2013;**23**:399-405

[67] Shams-White MM, Chung M, Du M, Fu Z, Insogna KL, Karlsen MC, et al. Dietary protein and bone health: A systematic review and meta-analysis from the National Osteoporosis Foundation. The American Journal of Clinical Nutrition. 2017;**105**:1528-1543

[68] Wu MJ, Chang CS, Cheng CH, Chen CH, Lee WC, Hsu YH, et al. Colonic transit time in long-term dialysis patients. American Journal of Kidney Diseases. 2004;**44**:322-327

[69] Roager HM, Hansen LB, Bahl MI, Frandsen HL, Carvalho V, Gobel RJ, et al. Colonic transit time is related to bacterial metabolism and mucosal turnover in the gut. Nature Microbiology. 2016;**1**:16093

Chapter 3

A New Dietary Therapy with Low Protein Processed Genmai (Brown Rice) for CKD by Correcting Gut-Kidney Axis

Shaw Watanabe, Shu Wakino, Yasushi Saiga, Katsuhiko Fukuda, Jun Mochizuki, Tan Wei, Qi Guo and Haerani Rasyid

Abstract

The number of chronic kidney disease (CKD) patients continues to increase globally, according to the increases in obesity, diabetes mellitus, hypertension, and aged people. When the glomerular lesions progress, it can lead to end-stage renal disease, which requires hemodialysis or transplantation. It is historically proven that a low-protein diet is effective for the palliative treatment of uremia. Current drug therapy targeting kidney lesions is insufficient, while dietary therapy is rather ignorant. We developed a low-protein processed genmai (brown rice) (LPPG) to improve CKD management. The essential functional features of brown rice are retained in LPPG and ameliorate the negative spiral of gut-kidney linkage caused by uremic dysbiosis and a leaky gut. LPPG is characterized by an energy value the same as white rice, a protein content of less than 0.2 g/100 g boiled rice, a potassium content that is almost zero, phosphorus of less than a quarter that of conventional rice, the presence of dietary fiber, γ-oryzanol, and antioxidant activity. We tried to clarify the functional mechanism to decrease uremic toxins by improvement of dysbiosis of the colonic microbiota, changes in short-chain fatty acids, and decreased uremic toxins and inflammatory biomarkers through pro- and post-intervention clinical trials in Japan, China, and Indonesia. Changes in microbiota were essential, with increased *Firmicutes* and decreased *Proteobacteria* at the phylum level, and *Blautia* played the essential role for gut microbiota reconstruction at the genus level. We propose a new personalized therapy with LPPG for all stages of CKD patients by decreasing uremic toxins and hidden inflammation.

Keywords: chronic kidney disease, dietary therapy, uremic toxin, microbiota, short-chain fatty acid (SCFA)

1. Introduction

Recent declarations by World Kidney Day sought to implement strategies that reduce the risk of renal failure by preventing CKD progression and controlling uremia without dialysis. Practical dietary interventions may have a role in improving CKD outcomes and preventing or delaying dialysis initiation [1].

We have studied a low-protein diet for CKD patients and succeeded in yielding the low-protein processed genmai (LPPG: JAS0027), *Gogyo-genmai,* to improve the bowel condition and decrease the uremic toxins [2]. Patients only replaced staple foods with LPPG without restricting side dishes, so it is easy to practice. We also developed the pro- and post-intervention study to provide evidence of the effects of LPPG [3].

Drug therapy for CKD has developed remarkably, but it cannot decrease the uremic toxins effectively [4, 5]. Our LPPG pack rice makes it easy to reduce protein, potassium (K), and phosphate (P) intake simultaneously and improves uremic dysbiosis and leaky gut by the water-insoluble dietary fiber, γ-oryzanol, and antioxidant activity.

Pro-post-intervention clinical trials of 1–9 months of LPPG intake reduced constipation due to increased acetic and propionic acid, recomposition by *Blautia,* and a decrease in potentially harmful bacteria, like *Escherichia coli*/Shigella. Decreased uremic toxins and inflammatory biomarkers, such as IL-6, sCRP, and TNFα, were also effective. Uremic toxins and inflammatory cytokines were factors promoting the CKD stage.

The intake of LPPG improved dysbiosis, changed SCFA, and decreased uremic toxins and inflammatory cytokines, resulting in improved clinical features. LPPG's low-protein diet is effective at all stages of CKD.

In this chapter, we will propose a new approach to personalized dietary therapy with LPPG.

2. Pathophysiology

There are various pathological conditions associated with kidney disease [6]. Still, in cases that do not heal, it progresses to chronic kidney disease, which may eventually progress into end-stage renal disease (ESRD), which requires dialysis or kidney transplantation. Therefore, despite the diversity of pathological diagnoses at onset, chronic cases are now diagnosed and treated collectively as chronic kidney disease (CKD). In the past, glomerulonephritis in childhood was a major cause, but recently, the proportion attributed to diabetes and hypertension, according to diabetes and aged people, has increased [4].

In diabetes, glycated substances form amyloid deposits in the glomeruli, leading to glomerular degeneration and sclerosis. Similarly, deposition by the immunoprecipitation mechanism is present in IgA nephropathy [7].

In hypertension, hyperfiltration causes dilation and hardening of the arterioles within the glomeruli, leading to the destruction of the pod cells and subsequent glomerular degeneration [8]. As the glomeruli degenerate and die, the peripherally connected tubules also undergo degeneration and disappearance, progressing to ultimate renal sclerosis (atrophic kidneys). Additionally, toxic substances in the tubules can cause degeneration and fibrosis, leading to upward glomerular degeneration. Recently, in Japan, puberulic acid poisoning from red yeast supplements affected the proximal tubules, presenting symptoms like Fanconi syndrome [9]. Several iatrogenic causes include aminoglycoside antibiotics, cisplatin and other anticancer agents, and radiographic contrast agents. Heavy metals, like cadmium, lead, and mercury, can also cause tubular degeneration [10].

A high-protein diet causes the formation of urea from deaminated nitrogen, which places a burden on the kidneys [11]. If uremia occurs, the intestinal microbiota changes to a proteobacteria-dominant one, and butyrate-producing bacteria decrease. Such changes alter the short-chain fatty acids (SCFA), metabolism, cytokine production, and intestinal immunity [12].

RenVanholder identified substances with high renal toxicity from a series of hemodialysis solutions and conceptualized them as uremic toxins (**Table 1**). Representative examples include cresyl sulfate, derived from phenols; indoxyl sulfate, derived from tryptophan; and phenyl sulfate, derived from phenylalanine. Metabolites such as kynurenine, methyl arginine, and inflammatory cytokines are also involved in uremic toxins. Uremic toxins produce free radicals, leading to mitochondrial dysfunction and cell death [13, 14].

Intestinal bacteria significantly influence the production of uremic toxins. Microcarbonate-based dialysis agents have been trying to remove uremic toxins, but the results are unsatisfactory [15, 16]. Attempts to suppress the production of uremic toxins by administering bacteria have been conducted in experimental animals, but no successful cases with probiotics have been reported in humans. We have noticed bacterial changes in CKD [2, 17–22].

These uremic toxins cause oxidative stress and inflammation in the kidneys, which accelerates the decline in renal function and disrupts the intestinal environment. For this reason, protein restriction is always recommended for CKD patients, but it restricts the selection of side dishes for each day, making it difficult to continue. In clinical practice, adherence to a low-protein diet is low. If we are too concerned about low protein, we will not be able to get enough energy, so enthusiasm for low-protein diet therapy is waning. There is a need to develop a new approach to diet therapy.

Inflammation stimulated by uremic toxins causes the release of cytokines such as IL6 and CRP from the liver, leading to systemic inflammation and causing further damage to the body's organs, including the heart, blood vessels, brain, and kidneys. As this gut-liver-kidney toxicity increases, it forms a negative spiral of the gut-kidney-cardiometabolic linkage. Unless this negative spiral is ameliorated, we cannot control CKD with drugs, such as antidiabetic drugs, hypertensive drugs, and diuretics that target the kidney (**Figure 1**).

p-cresyl sulfate
Phenyl sulfate
Indoxyl sulfate
Symetric and Asymmetric dimethyl arginine
Kynurenines
Carbamylated compounds
Beta2 microglobulin
IL-6
TNFalpha
AGEs

Table 1.
Uremic toxins with the highest evidence score (4) by Vanholder.

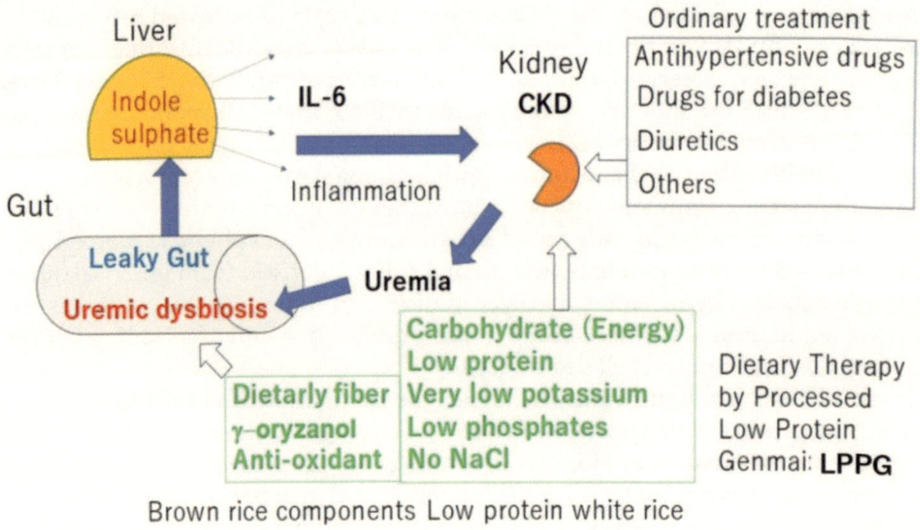

Figure 1.
The gut-kidney negative spiral and the target of LPPG.

3. Drug therapy of CKD according to the guidelines

The guidelines employ drug therapies tailored to the causes of CKD [23]. These include hypoglycemic agents for diabetes, antihypertensive agents for hypertension, antibiotics for inflammation, and diuretics for edema. However, a recent trend has shifted from uniform guideline-based treatment to tailored individualized medicine. Nevertheless, dietary therapy does not carry much weight, probably due to the varying effects demonstrated in randomized clinical studies. As a result, physicians tend to focus on drug therapy.

The Kidney Disease: Improving Global Outcomes (KDIGO) 2024 and the Japanese Society of Nephrology guidelines 2023 editions for drug therapy have undergone several significant changes (**Table 2**).

Blood pressure control is significant but incomplete for renal protection. Albuminuria, urinary protein, high triglycerides, and low HDL cholesterol are strong independent predictors of CKD onset in diabetes. The long-term intraindividual variation in HbA1c, blood pressure, lipid parameters, and uric acid plays a greater role in the progression of CKD than the absolute value of each single variable [24, 25].

A recent rapid expansion of treatment options includes sodium-glucose co-transporter-2 inhibitors (SGLT2i), nonsteroidal mineralocorticoid receptor antagonists, and glucagon-like peptide-1 receptor agonists [26].

The use of SGLT2 inhibitors has expanded indications beyond diabetic nephropathy to nondiabetic kidney diseases by inhibiting CKD progression and reducing cardiovascular risk. However, its effectiveness is limited to obese people, so similar effects would be seen with fasting or obesity control by a low-calorie diet and exercise to decrease body weight.

Low bone mineral density is associated with a risk of fractures even in patients with CKD in the maintenance phase. The 2017 revised KDIGO chronic kidney disease mineral and bone disorder (CKD-MBD) guidelines propose including bone mineral density as a clinical indicator. Balanced minerals in brown rice are comparative, as described later.

	Proteinuria (+)		Proteinuria (−)
CKD stage	1st selection	ACE inhibitor, ARB	ACE inhibitor, ARB
G1-G3		Ca antagonist	Ca antagonist
		Thiazide diuretics	Thiazide diuretics
G4,G5		ACE inhibitor, ARB	ACE inhibitor, ARB
		Ca antagonist	Ca antagonist
		Roop diuretics	Roop diuretics
G4, G5	1st selection	ACE inhibitor, ARB	
		beta blocker	
		MRA	
		SGL2 inhibitor	
		ARNI	
		Ivabrajin	

ACE: angiotensin-converting enzyme; ARB:angiotensin II receptor blocker; CKD: chronic kidney disease; MRA: mineralcorticoid receptor antagonist; SGL: sodium glucose co-tansporter 2.

Table 2.
Recommendation of antihypertensive agents for heart failure in patients with CKD.

An individualized risk assessment, "The Kidney Failure Risk Equation," recommends treatment plans based on individual patient risk [27].

4. Dietary therapy

4.1 Low-protein processed brown rice

Unpolished brown rice contains many functional components and has significant health benefits [28]. In the past, low-protein white rice lost the bran layer, which includes most functional components. Brown rice contains six times more dietary fiber than white rice and is rich in minerals and vitamins [29].

Grains are covered by a strong wax layer, preventing protein-degrading enzyme solutions from penetrating. Additionally, aerobic spores and other bacteria contaminate the surface of the grains. We selected organic rice varieties, performed appropriate grain surface treatment, chose an enzyme solution to break down rice protein, and cooked 100 g portions of deproteinized brown rice in steam for 10 minutes [30]. After cooking, we sealed the rice under high-temperature conditions. The Ministry of Agriculture, Forestry, and Fisheries approved LPPG as JAS0027 (**Table 3**).

Each pack of PLLG contains 150 g of protein-deleted brown rice with a protein content of 0.3 g. Patients who consume three meals daily can ingest 700 kcal, but the protein content is only 0.9 g. Minerals remain: potassium, which is deleted by more than 95%, and phosphorus, which is removed by three-quarters, with no NaCl. Gamma oryzanol and antioxidants express various functions along the gut-brain axis. LPPG's antioxidant activity maintains 1350 mmol TEQeq, which provides one-fourth of the recommended daily dose [31].

Nutrients of LPPG (Gogyo-genmai)	Brawn Rice*	LPPG*	Gogyo-genmai**
Energy (kcal)	244	156	234
Water (g)	40.7	62.2	93.3
Protein (g)	1.3	0.2	0.3
Lipid (g)	1.9	1.3	1.95
Ash (g)	0.1	0.1	0.15
Carbohydrate (g)	57.1	36.3	54.45
Sugar (g)	55.6	35.3	52.95
Dietary fiber (g)	1.5	1.0	1.5
γ-oryzanol (mg)	10.4	6.3	9.45
Sodium (mg)	2.5	1.2	1.8
NaCleq (g)	0.0041	0.003	0.0045
K (mg)	85.3	0.5	0.75
P (mg)	115	14.8	22.2
Ca (mg)	6	6	9
Mg (mg)	47.5	2.2	3.3
Mn (mg)	0.83	0.05	0.075
Zn (mg)	0.76	0.12	0.18
Fe (mg)	0.4	<0.1	<0.1
Cu (mg)	0.1	<0.1	<0.1

**means/100 g boiled rice.*
***means/per package (150 g).*

Table 3.
Nutrients in the brown rice and low-protein processed Genmai.

4.2 Genmai and microbiota in healthy people

Brown rice contains a lot of insoluble dietary fiber, so a large amount reaches the large intestine, serving as nutrition for bacteria [32].

An increase in the number of medications administered caused a decrease in the diversity of bacterial species. Many of these bacteria produce SCFAs, such as butyrate and acetate. These are *Blautia, Facaebacterium, Lachnospiraceae, Eubacterium, Clostridium,* and *Dorea* [33].

Many healthy people run a brown rice-based vegetarian diet in groups such as the Japan Society of Integrative Medicine, the Japan CI Association, the Japan Macrobiotic Association, and the AOB KEIO Group [34]. Most of them have the same root as Sagen Ishizuka [35]. We found that the *genmai* (brown rice) eaters were healthy, not obese, and had good bowel conditions. We considered that the intestinal microbiota would have a key role and planned to perform the nested study on intestinal microbiota among the participants in the GENKI study [36]. One thousand two hundred twenty-two people from all over Japan had been involved and reported their contribution to the health benefits of the brown rice diet. A questionnaire survey was conducted for a person who participated in GENKI study I for the second time 1 year later, and we obtained 350 respondents.

One hundred nine healthy subjects (18 males and 90 females) provided stools for analysis. The average age was 53 years old, and the BMIs of both sexes were 22.1 ± 3.2 in males and 20.7 ± 2.8 in females, respectively.

Bacterial profiles at phylum level were as follows; *Firmicutes* 44.3 ± 9.9%, *Bacteroides* 20.7 ± 8.8%, *Actinobacteria* 8.3 ± 6.3%, *Proteobacteria* 1.7 ± 2.7%, and *Verrucobacteria* 1.2 ± 4.2% (max 39.4%). Brown rice eaters showed additional benefits due to the high prevalence of *Firmicutes* and low prevalence of *Fusobacterium*. Habitual rice eaters showed *a dominant Faecalibacterium and Blautia* profile of intestinal microbiota [21].

Then we conducted an intervention study in which participants consumed a genmai rice cake (*omusubi*) five times a week for lunch for 12 weeks as part of a trial by the Ministry of Agriculture, Forestry, and Fisheries [22]. We implemented a simple food-based guideline for taking side dishes [37]. After 3 months, approximately half of the participants experienced weight loss, and bowel movements and stool consistency improved significantly—the intestinal microbiota altered SCFA production. The genmai diet increased stable butyrate-producing bacteria, stimulated the proliferation of regulatory T cells, and enhanced natural immunity.

Predominant microbiota were *Firmicutes* (around 65%), *Actinobacteria* (15–17%), *Bacteroides* (5–7%), and less than 1% of *Proteobacteria*, *Verrucomicrobia*, *Fusobacteria*, and rare *Synergistetes* and *Euryarchaeota*. In SCFA, acetate and propionate tended to decrease, while n-butyrate and i-valerate increased.

Acetate, propionate, n-butyrate, and n-valerate had positive correlations with IL-6, and n-butyrate, i-butyrate, and n-valerate showed positive correlations with CRP. These SCFAs did not have correlations with TNF-α.

About 40% of the subjects succeeded in improving their microbiota profile and bowel movement, with good stool condition, by simply changing lunch to brown rice balls (onigiri) 5 days a week.

4.3 Rationale of the LPPG intervention study for CKD patients

CKD is diagnosed based on abnormalities in urine analysis and a decline in kidney function. As patients' quality of life declined, soaring medical costs and the burden of care associated with hospital visits and home stays have become a robust social problem [38].

CKD progresses due to the accumulation of risk factors, such as high blood pressure, impaired glucose tolerance, and obesity, and the management of lifestyle-related diseases is essential for suppressing its progression.

Diet therapy is a part of everyday life, so not only doctors and nutritionists, who are outsiders, but even the people themselves cannot see it. There is a strong perception that diet therapy is a supplementary treatment in the medical field, and medical personnel's sense of responsibility is relatively weak [39]. Placement of controls is an essential condition in RCTs; however, feeding a placebo diet for a long time is not possible in dietary therapy.

We developed an epidemiological strategy for pro- and post-design [3]. We devised a design to reduce protein intake by changing the staple food without setting a standard point, as past clinical trials could not adhere to the standard for low-protein diets.

Previous RCTs' results often exceeded the guided amount for actual protein intake. In the Northern Italian Multi-Center Trial, the set instruction amount was 0.6 g/kg BW/day from the beginning but became 0.846 g/kg BW/day, a 39.8% excess at the end.

In the MDRD study, doctors recommended the low-protein diet group (LPD) take 0.58 g/kg BW/day, but the actual intake was 0.72 g/kg BW/day. In the MDRD study, despite the initially required energy intake being 35 kal/kg BW/day, the average energy intake of subjects was about 25 kal/kg BW/day in the end [40]. Thus, almost all RCTs of dietary therapy failed due to the difficulty in keeping the programmed amount of protein and energy source intake throughout the study period [3].

Intervention trials with control groups may initially seem scientific and good, but they are challenging to implement. When we consider the level of intestinal bacteria, it is impossible to select control subjects who are equivalent to the intervention group. Even in crossover trials, if one side gets good results, it pulls the control subjects toward that side, so it is impossible to carry out the study as designed. Although the pro- and post-comparison studies often seem biased, we can examine the effects rationally if biomarkers are present appropriately.

Above all, general practitioners can easily conduct intervention studies even with a small number of participants (10 people or less), and they are inexpensive compared to RCTs. Considering it a series of case studies, we can also use them in personalized medicine. The food industry cannot afford the high costs of RCTs like the pharmaceutical industry, so unless they change their approach, they will not be able to improve the level of evidence.

For most practitioners, pro- and post-test comparison also benefits cost, ease of practice, and comprehensiveness [3]. The main weakness of the pro- and post-test design is that it cannot detect other possible causes of positive or negative results among the participants. Specific biomarkers give us insight into avoiding confounding factors.

4.4 Clinical intervention study by pro- and post-comparison design

Appropriate introduction and dietary guidelines assist individuals seeking to manage or improve their health. The study plan was approved by the Medical Station Clinic Ethics Review Committee and each institution. Low-protein processed genmai (JAS0027) improved the negative spiral of the gut-kidney axis caused by uremic dysbiosis and leaky gut [2, 41]. Replacing the main staple with an LPPG, while not strictly restricting side dishes, makes it easy to lower protein intake. Additionally, making meals tasty is a crucial factor for long-term adherence. Under a solution-oriented strategy, maintaining good adherence to low-protein intake is achievable.

LPPG is thought to be effective in reducing renal toxins from the pre-disease state of CKD to the dialysis stage, and we have conducted intervention studies to cover the range from CKD 2–5, depending on the facility (**Figure 2**). We also considered the geographical difference of the study area [42].

The research design was to eat the LPPG rice pack as a staple food twice daily, 5 days a week, with no other restrictions. Before and after the experiment, we measured the intestinal microbiota, SCFA, urinary protein, blood urea, and kidney function.

We measured plasma uremic toxins, sIgA, and inflammatory cytokines. We decided to evaluate the effects by resolving intestinal bacteria's dysbiosis and reducing uremic toxins and urinary proteins, simplifying the overall research.

We implemented the same protocol in Tianjin and Nanjing in China and Hasanuddin University in Indonesia. Would it be effective for Chinese and Indonesians, whose intestinal flora would differ? To conduct clinical trials overseas, we standardized the research design as much as possible. The Ministry of Agriculture, Forestry, and Fisheries supported the research by the BRIDGE fund. The conductors

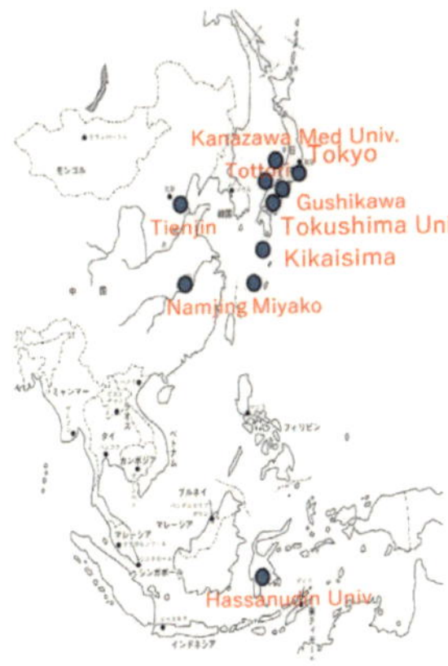

Study areas and number of participants in Dietary Therapy for CKD by Gogyognmai.
All show good bowel movement, and proteinuria ameliorates 40-50%. No racial difference.

	G0	G1	G2	G3a	G3b	G4	G5	Total
Tokyo	15	1	3	4	5	4	1	33
Kikaisima	6	1	5	1				13
Miyako			13	4	4		1	22
Tokushima				5	5	8	1	19
Kanazawa					1	4	3	8
Tottori	3				2			5
Kisiwada					1	2	6	9
Nanjing		23	2	4	3			32
Tianjin				4		4	2	10
Hassnudin			1	2	5	17	6	31
Total	24	25	24	18	21	35	18	182

Figure 2.
Study area and number of participants in the dietary therapy for CKD by LPPG.

were presented at the 2nd and 3rd International Workshop on Dietary Therapy for CKD, which was held in Okinawa in March 2024 and 2025 [39, 41].

4.5 Administration route, dosage, and administration period

We targeted patients with CKD stage G3 or lower who were attending the nephrology department and had not yet received nutritional therapy. We also called healthy volunteers for comparison. Since regular hospital visits are usually carried out every 3 months, a three-month intervention period was considered appropriate to minimize the burden on patients due to hospital visits.

After receiving nutritional guidance for LPPG as outpatients, the participants switched the main meal to LPPG. Specifically, for 5 days a week, LPPG was consumed instead of the usual main meal. Record how many packs the patient has consumed per week to check compliance. However, on the 2 days when the participants did not eat the LPPG pack, eating the usual main meal (white rice, bread, noodles, etc.) within the range that adhered to the daily protein intake was permissible.

Food guidelines for side dishes are based on the three-color food guide [37]. The mnemonic phrase "ma-go-ta-chi-wa-ya-sa-si-i," which means "grandchildren are kind," promotes the intake of specific foods for side dishes, such as beans, sesame seeds, eggs, milk, vegetables, fish, mushrooms, and potatoes (taro). Plant-based food guidelines show a similar pattern [43–45].

CKD patients follow two dietary guidelines using an LPPG pack. First, they consume 0.4 units of energy per kilogram of body weight. One unit equals 80 kcal, which aligns with the Japanese Diabetes Society's food exchange table. 0.4 units equate to 32 kcal, consistent with the 30–35 kcal guideline. One LPPG pack contains 2.25 mg of potassium, 76.5 mg of phosphorus, and low detectable sodium chloride. Dietary fiber is 4.5 g, and γ-oryzanol is 28.4 mg, which are expected to stabilize the intestinal microbiota and ecosystem. Antioxidant capacity is 300 μmol TEQ, which is also likely to be effective [46, 47].

When the protein intake from each side dish is approximately 10 grams (about 50 grams of meat or fish), this constitutes a low-protein diet while still allowing patients to eat foods like those of their family.

No special side dishes are specified, but animal meat and fish should be limited to about 50 g per meal (about one egg). Vegetable proteins (tofu, natto, etc.) were good [37, 44–46]. Salt should be kept to a minimum (about 6 g per day), especially for those with high blood pressure. Aerobic exercise was good at any CKD stage.

To confirm the effects of a low-protein diet, it is advisable to check for protein in urine. Urinary protein is a simple and accurate prognostic indicator that can motivate patients. In a 10-year follow-up study of 40,000 healthy individuals in Okinawa, a simple urine test using a test strip indicated the risk of progressing to end-stage disease [48].

5. Effects of LPPG low-protein diet

5.1 Study areas and outline of participants

Figure 2 shows participants in the study area and the degree of CKD (**Figure 2**).

In Tokyo, participants voluntarily participated in the study. In Kikaigashima and Miyako, participants came from the local health check-up screening program. In Kanazawa, Tokushima, and Kishiwada, patients in advanced CKD stages are treated in the nephrology department of the university or a specific hospital. In the case of Shimane Integrative Medicine Center, the patients developed CKD as a COVID-19 infection or vaccine complication. In China and Indonesia, the participants are patients in nephrology-specific hospitals or clinics.

Dietary habits in these areas, as shown by the chief component analysis of FFF data, were not so different, although people in Tokyo tended to eat Japanese-style foods, and in Miyako, more Westernized foods like bread, coffee, chicken, egg, milk, and meat were preferred [42].

The number of participants and their CKD stage are shown in the table (**Figure 2**).

The average age was the sixties. In Miyako, long-term intake of LPPG for up to 9 months was carried out to see the intestinal stability and safety. Age was related to the CKD stage, and most patients taking LPPG for more than 6 months came from Miyako (**Figure 2**).

The mean age of the 32 participants in the Nanjing study (15 males and 17 females) was 62.1 ± 16.1 years. Sixteen had diabetes, five had hypertension, one had diabetes plus hypertension, one was obese, and 25 had CKD stages 1–2, 3 had 3a, and 4 had 3b, most in the early stage. Urine protein was + in 19 and ± in 9. After 3 months of LPPG intake, + was in 5, ± in 10, and - in 16; 50.6% improved. eGFR also improved in half of the patients, as did IL-6. Tianjin was mainly CKD4, and bowel movements and blood urea improved in this 1-month intervention trial. Hasanudein University in Indonesia included 32 CKD patients, 18 males and 14 females, with positive urinary protein. The mean age was 58.4 ± 11.3 years, and CKD stage was CKD 4 in 21 patients, 3 in 7 patients, and 5 in 6 patients. After 1 month of intervention, there was an improvement in bowel movements, an increase in propionic acid, and a significant decrease in Cr ($p = 0.01$).

5.2 Clinical findings after LPPG intervention trial in Japan

The earliest clinical finding was the resolution of constipation. The compliance rate of LPPG packs was more than 95% in all areas. Body weight decreased, blood pressure ameliorated, and blood glucose and creatinine decreased (**Table 4**). The decrease of glomerular filtration rates in both creatinine and cysteine-based GFR was not worsened but improved.

		Pro			Post			
		mean		sd	mean		sd	p
Age	year	70.32	±	7.54				
Body weight	kg	68.57	±	13.22	68.09	±	12.73	0.17
BMI	kg/m^2	25.87	±	4.04	25.69	±	4.03	0.22
systolic BP	mmHg	138.16	±	12.62	132.26	±	14.78	0.03
diastolic BP	mmHg	83.95	±	12.00	78.53	±	14.22	0.03
Protein intake/day	g/day	53.04	±	19.7	51.94	±	18.92	0.31
Protein intake/kgbw	g/kgbw	0.89	±	0.28	0.88	±	0.29	0.31
BUN	mg/dl	23.26	±	9.06	22.00	±	7.52	0.29
Creatinine	mg/dl	1.84	±	1.14	1.78	±	1.11	<0.001
eGFR	ml/min/1.73m^2	32.84	±	11.36	34.42	±	12.75	0.03
Cr clearance*	ml/min/1.73m^2	51.32	±	23.48	52.78	±	24.72	<0.001
Salt intake/day	g/day	9.36	±	3.26	7.92	±	2.82	0.03
sCRP	mg/dl	0.30	±	0.81	0.10	±	0.11	0.44
IL-6	pg/ml	4.66	±	4.82	2.76	±	0.97	0.03
TNFα	pg/ml	12.17	±	3.26	11.59	±	2.74	0.46
Phenyl Sulfate	ug/ml	2.65	±	2.09	2.75	±	2.64	0.57
Paracresyl Sulfate	ug/ml	8.77	±	5.35	5.47	±	4.49	0.03
Indoxyl Sulfate	ug/ml	3.26	±	3.31	3.22	±	2.98	0.96

**Calculation of sCRP: males: (140-age)*body weight/(72*Cr); females: 0.85*(140-age)*body weight/(72*Cr).*

Table 4.
Effects of LPPG interventions. pro- and post-comparison in Tokushima and Kishiwada.

The patients continued taking the packs for 6–9 months without problems. The patients' comments were mostly positive, saying that the food was delicious and easy to eat, that they did not feel forced to change their staple food, that there were few restrictions on side dishes, and that they enjoyed their new diet with family. The protein intake was generally less than 0.8 g/kg, and some became 0.5 g/kg. Reduction in urinary protein was seen in about half of the patients. This effect was also seen in patients with relatively advanced CKD (stages 4–5).

The amount of urinary toxins in each stage of CKD was lower in patients in stage 3a for phenyl sulfate and paracresyl sulfate; still, there was no apparent difference for indoxyl sulfate. The levels increased with each stage of advanced CKD. Looking at the dynamics of inflammatory markers in patients in stages 3 and above, CRP decreased in stages 3a and 3b but increased in stages 4 and 5. IL6 decreased in stages 3a and 5 but increased in stages 3b and 4. TNFα increased in all stages.

Table 4 shows the changes in BMI, blood pressure, and the changes in urinary protein, protein intake, BUN, creatinine, and eGFR for 30 cases from Tokushima University and Kishiwada Hospital. We also compared changes in inflammatory biomarkers such as UPCR, CRP, IL-6, and TNF-alpha, and changes in urinary toxins such as phenyl sulfate, paracresyl sulfate, and indoxyl sulfate. All indicators improved except urine protein, albumin, Ccr, and TNFα in 3b; eGFR was maintained or slightly improved. All three types of urinary toxins decreased in stage 4.

5.3 Changes in microbiota

Comparison of microbiota at baseline (Pro) and 3 months later (post) showed an increase in *Firmicutes* and a decrease in *Proteobacteria, Bacteroidetes*, and *Euryarchaeota* at the phylum level. *Actinobacteria* and *Verrucomicrobia* slightly decreased (**Table 5**).

The 25 bacterial species accounted for 1% or more. It does not take into account the stage of CKD. *Blautia wexlerae, Fusicatenibacteer saccharovorans, and Collincela aerofacience increased at the species level. Blautia wexlerae* was the most abundant species. *Bifidobacterium adolescentis* and *Bifidobacterium catenulatum* decreased with disease progression. *E. coli/Shigella* increased as the disease progressed, reaching a maximum of 22%.

Chief component analysis showed *Blautia* species scattered in five factors at baseline,

In the post-intervention state, butyrate-producing bacteria like *Clostridium* occupied the first factor, so-called bad bacilli, *like Escherichia colli/Shigella* in the second factor, *Blautia hommnis/hansenii* belonged to the 3rd factor with *Streptococcus* and *Enterococcus. 4th and 5th were Bacteroides and Bifidobacterium (negative). Blautia wexlerae* is present in the 6th factor with butyric acid-producing bacilli, like *Butylicococcus faecihomins, Dialister hominins, Geniner homicides*, and *Slackia isoflavoconverta* (**Figure 3**).

The correlation between each bacterium in pro is only a few for *Blautia wexlerae.* At the same time, *Blautia sps*. Are distributed across six factors, with some bacteria showing positive and negative relationships within each factor. However, in the post state, *Blautia spp*. disperse into six factors and show strong positive correlations with other bacteria in each factor. The number of bacteria in the same factor shows only positive relationships with Blautia spp.

Bifidobacterium adolescentis and *Bifidobacterium catenulatum* decreased with disease progression.

In the post state, *Blautia wexlera*e shows significant correlations with many bacteria, such as *Bifidobacterium catenulatum* (CC = .909**), *Anaerobutyricum hallii* (CC = .914**), *Streptococcus lactarius* (937**), C*ollinsella aerofaciens* (CC = .722**), *Streptococcus salivarius* (CC = .775**), *Bifidobacterium*

	Pro			Post			
Phylum	**mean (%)**		**sd**	**mean (%)**		**sd**	**p**
Firmicutes	57.637	±	13.934	60.847	±	18.806	0.158
Actinobacteria	33.527	±	15.641	33.747	±	20.302	0.875
Proteobacteria	2.556	±	7.280	0.489	±	1.13	0.14
Verrucomicrobia	0.661	±	2.305	0.510	±	1.961	0.79
Bacteroidetes	0.247	±	0.417	0.095	±	0.144	0.638
Euryarchaeota	0.178	±	0.703	0.102	±	0.402	0.068
Fusobacteria	0.001	±	0.002	0.002	±	0.006	0.317
Synergistetes	0.011	±	0.032	0.000	±	0.000	

Table 5.
Changes in microbiota at the phylum level in pro and post stage.

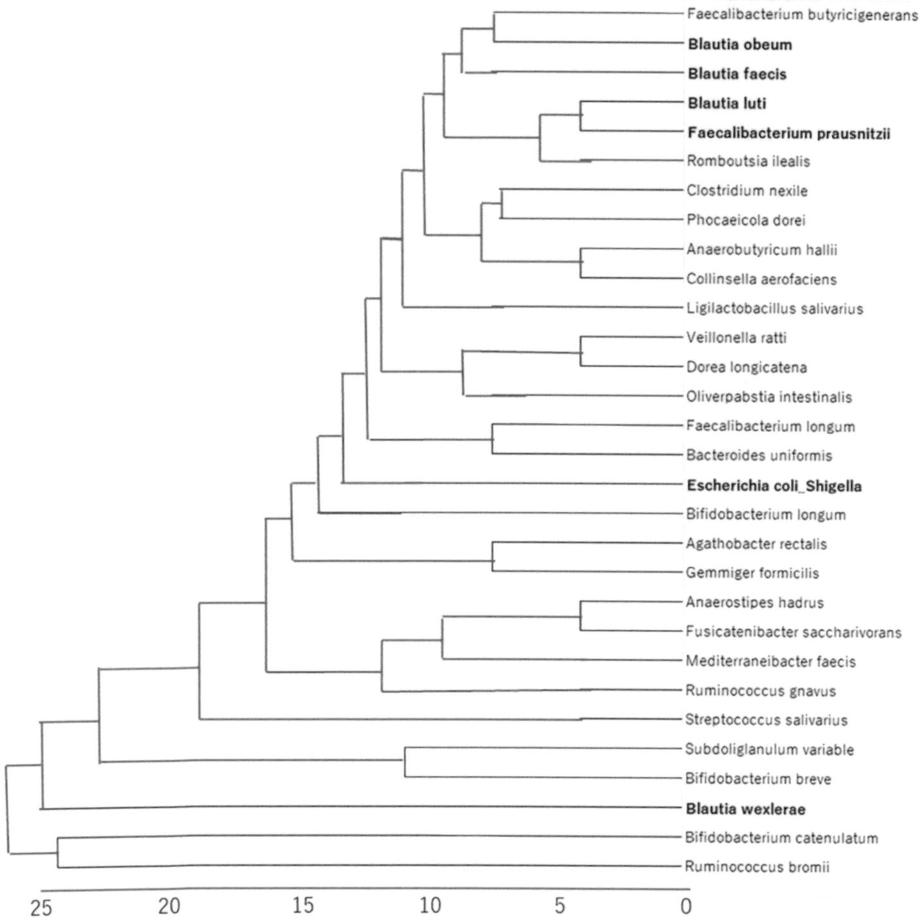

Figure 3.
Cluster analysis, which shows correlations between these bacilli. Cluster dendrogram of species showing independence of Blautia wexlerae.

longum (CC = .746**), *Blautia obeum* (CC = .672**), and *Bifidobacterium bifidum* (CC = .649**), *Gemmiger formicilis* (CC = .622**), *Fusicatenibacter saccharivorans* (CC = .512**), *Mediterraneibacter faecis* (CC = .636**), *Ruminococcus bromii* (CC = .365*), *Blautia faecis* (.637**), *Bifidobacterium bifidum* (.649**), *Gemmiger formicilis* (.622**), *Dorea formicigenerans* (.637**), *Streptococcus anginosus* (.647**), *Catenibacterium mitsuokai* (.635**), *Ligilactobacillus salivarius* (.529**), *Lacticaseibacillus casei* (.491**), *Streptococcus sinensis* (.648**), *Eubacterium coprostanoligenes* (.656**), *Terrisporobacter petrolearius* (.853**), *Enterococcus asini* (.753**), *Clostridium perfringens* (.636**), *Hespellia porcina* (.636**), *Coprococcus catus* (.636**), *Eubacterium callanderi* (.647**), Bifidobacterium breve (.636**), *Murimonas intestine* (.695**), *Lactococcus lactis* (.636**), *Blautia hominis* (.684**), *Thermophilibacter provencensis* (.699**), *Tractidigestivibacter scatoligenes* (.647**), *Blautia faecicola* (.642**), *Blautia faecis* (CC = 637**), and *Lachnospira eligens2* (.629**) *$p<0.05$, **$p<0.01$.

This can be explained by the idea that *Blautia wexlerae* controls other *Blautia* species and regulates the overall gut microbiota society. In the post state, Shannon's diversity also increased, suggesting a return to a normal state from a dysbiosis state.

5.4 Changes of SCFA

sIgA and SCFA in Pro- and Post phase are shown in **Table 6**.

Acetate correlated with propionic acid (CC = .598**) and n-butyric acid (CC = .723**), and propionic acid correlated with n-butyrate (CC = .505**), i-butyrate (CC = .421*), n-valeric acid (CC = 433*), and i-valeric acid (CC = 447**). Furthermore, i-valeric acid strongly correlated with n-valeric acid (CC = .744**).

Succinic acid showed a correlation only with isovaleric acid (CC = 386*).

Butyrate is crucial as it provides an energy source for epithelial cells and plays a significant physiological role [49–53]. Major butyrate producers in the human gut are *Faecalibacterium prausnitzii, Eubacterium rectale, Eubacterium hallii, Ruminococcus bromii, Butyricicoccus pullicaecorum, Roseburia spp.*, and *Anaerostipes spp*.

All bacteria belonged to the phylum *Firmicutes*. Their genomes are crucial for dietary fiber digestion and butyrate production, but have a lower proportion of genes for inulin utilization and propionate production.

When looking at the relationship between sIgA and SCFA as an indicator of intestinal immunity, there was no significant correlation between sIgA and SCFA. However, there was a correlation with specific bacteria. The two most dominant bacterial species with a significant contribution to butyrate production in the human colon are *Faecalibacterium prausnitzii* in clusters IV and *Eubacterium rectale* in cluster XIVa [22].

5.5 Changes of uremic toxins and inflammation markers

In recent years, it has become known that chronic inflammation in CKD patients is associated with the progression of CKD, protein-energy wasting, and mortality [53]. The Chronic Renal Insufficiency Cohort study demonstrated that biomarkers of inflammation are related to renal function. It has also been reported that the cause of increased blood cytokine levels is not only due to the kidney's decline in excretion function but also due to the effects of the underlying disease and diet. The impact of intestinal flora on uremic toxins has been suggested as a cause of increased

	Pro				Post			
	mean		sd	median	mean		sd	median
sIgA	1156.39	±	1247.97	**789.65**	1197.32	±	1815.03	**504.50**
succinate	0.41	±	0.50	0.21	0.89	±	1.42	0.40
lactate	0.36	±	0.37	0.23	1.07	±	1.49	0.46
formate	0.17	±	0.11	0.13	0.11	±	0.01	0.11
acetate	4.07	±	1.80	**4.06**	4.92	±	2.76	**4.46**
proprionate	1.56	±	0.80	1.45	1.79	±	1.09	1.40
iso-butyrate	0.21	±	0.08	0.20	0.16	±	0.07	0.12
n-butyrate	1.00	±	0.67	**0.73**	1.47	±	1.31	**1.50**
i-valerate	0.38	±	0.19	0.34	0.26	±	0.17	0.22
n-valerate	0.34	±	0.16	0.34	0.33	±	0.15	0.31

Table 6.
Median of sIgA decreased at the post-phase, probably due to the sedation of inflammation. Succinate, lactate, acetate and n-butyrate increased among SCFA.

inflammatory cytokine production, and in patients with CKD stages 3–4, renal and cardiovascular toxins (indoxyl sulfate and p-cresyl sulfate) produced only by intestinal bacteria have been shown to increase.

In recent years, it has become known that chronic inflammation in CKD patients is associated with the progression of CKD, protein-energy wasting, and mortality. The Chronic Renal Insufficiency Cohort study (CRIC study) demonstrated that inflammatory biomarkers (IL-1β, IL-1 receptor antagonist, IL-6, TNF-α, CRP, and fibrinogen) are inversely correlated with eGFR [54]. These relationships have been summarized and are now attracting attention as the "kidney-gut axis" or "intestinal-renal axis."

Salt restriction is currently the recommended dietary therapy for CKD, and little guidance has been provided on protein restriction.

5.6 Interaction between bacteria, SCFA, and sIgA

sIgA, an indicator of intestinal immunity, did not significantly correlate with any SCFAs. sIgA was mainly around 2000 mg/g feces, but when it was low, it was around 500 mg; when it was high, it was over 5000 mg. Five people out of 200 (2.5%) always had only a two-digit amount. One of them was using methotrexate for rheumatoid arthritis. There were no cases of complete absence.

When a cluster dendrogram is made using sIgA, SCFA, renal toxins, and inflammatory markers as variables, the results are divided into three clusters (**Figure 4**). The center forms a cluster with paracresylS and IL6, indoxylS and CKD stage, and phenyl S and TNFα, and the final cluster is formed by overlapping acetic acid, propionic acid, and acetic acid, n-butyric acid, and n-valeric acid, and sCRP. The only significant factors forming the CKD stage progression were all three uremic toxins and IL6, TNFα.

The cluster dendrogram made from negative correlations shows a negative pair;

N-butyrate and TNFα, phenyl sulfate and sCRP, lactate and progression of CKD, SIgA and IL-6, propronate and paracresyl sulfate, and acetate and indoxyl sulfate, suggest the cross relationship that decreased SCFA increases uremic toxins.

The balance between the decreased SCFA and increased uremic toxins explains the pathology of dysbiosis.

sIgA showed a positive correlation with *Bifidobacterium catenulatum* (CC = .309*) and *Escherichia coli* (CC = .324*) (**Table 7**). In many cases where LPPG was consumed for 1 month, there was a tendency for sIgA to decrease. The relationship between SCFA and bacteria was observed with a correlation between acetate and *Blautia wexlerae* (CC = .311*) and succinate and *Blautia faecis* (CC = .553*). Lactic acid consistently showed a strong correlation with *Bifidobacterium adolescentis* (CC = 961**), *Ruminococcus gnavus* (CC = .933*), *Doria longicatena* (CC = .949*), and *Romboutsia ilealis* (CC = 985**). Additionally, propionate significantly correlated with *Akkermansia muciniphila* (CC = .394**) and n-butyrate with *Agathobacter rectalis* (CC = .355*). The relationship between *Blautia wexlerae* and acetate was a common finding among brown rice eaters [21, 22]. In groups with high acetate, the proportion of *Blautia wexlerae* often accounted for 10–20%.

Recovery from uremic dysbiosis started from the lowered pH in the colon, which suppresses the growth of proteobacteria, like *E. coli*, and *Blautia wexlerae* conducted to recovery of microflora with *Phecobacterium prausnizii* for butyrate-producing bacteria.

Akkermansia showed a strong positive correlation with E. coli (CC = .534**) and a strong correlation with *Gemminger formicilis* (CC = .715**). Although various

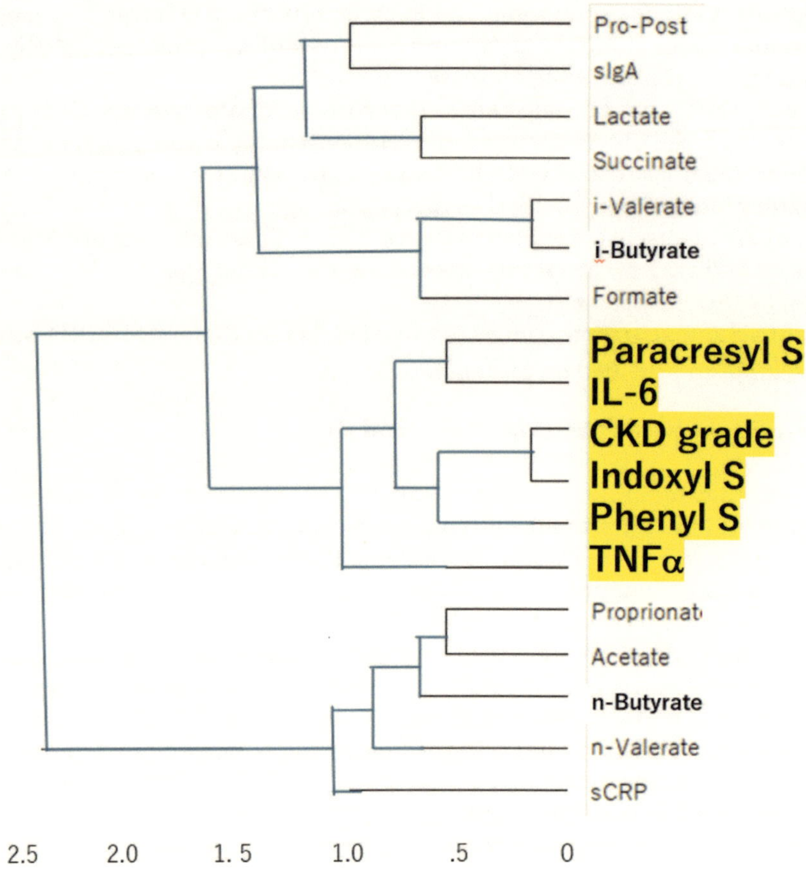

Figure 4.
Cluster dendrogram of Positive correlation among CKD grade, SCFA and inflammation markers. CKD progression (CKD grade) is clustered among uremic toxins and inflammation markers (IL-6 and TNFα).

interactions between *Akkermansia* and different bacteria have been reported experimentally, they are not necessarily beneficial, even if they are present on mucosal surfaces in humans. Propionate correlated with *Akkermansia* (**Table** 7 and **Figure** 5)

6. Proposal for the future

Until the 1960s, dietary therapy was the only treatment for uremia [55]. Vohlhard successfully reduced uremia with a starch diet in 1918, and subsequently, Giordano, Grovannetti and others achieved better results by ensuring adequate energy intake and considering amino acid scores.

Uremic toxins, mainly coming from amino acids, always worsen renal damage at any CKD grade. A high-protein diet increases uremic toxins, potassium, and phosphorus accumulation, worsens acidosis, and worsens kidney function. As a new approach, the KDOQI CPG 2012 recommends sodium, potassium, phosphorus, and protein restriction, and the KDOQI 2020 guideline recommends a low-protein diet of 0.55–0.6 g/kg body weight/day [56].

Additionally, the PLADO diet is recommended, which improves the intestinal environment through dietary fiber, alleviates acidosis with potassium-rich fruits and

DOI: http://dx.doi.org/10.5772/intechopen.1011052

	sIgA	Bautia wexlerae	Bifidobact. catenulatum[1]	Bifidobact. adolescentis	Ruminococcus gravus	Agathbactor rectalis	Escherichia coli/Shigela	Bulatia faecis	Dorea longicatena	Romboutsia iealis	Akkermancia muciniphila
sIgA	1	0.101	**.309***	−0.169	−0.084	0.141	**.324***	0.126	0.136	−0.022	0.207
Succinate	−0.028	0.055	−0.156	−0.125	−0.09	−0.072	−0.065	**.553****	−0.16	−0.063	−0.042
Lactate	0.103	0.514	−0.23	**.961****	**.933***	−0.333	−0.299	−0.802	**.949***	**.985****	−0.300
Acetate	0.217	**.311***	0.031	−0.083	0.137	**.340***	−0.156	−0.077	0.277	**.381***	−0.154
Propionate	0.187	0.173	−0.145	−0.143	0.12	0.241	0.261	−0.152	0.190	0.130	**.394****
i-butyrate	0.043	0.126	0.056	−0.308	0.08	0.027	−0.018	−0.018	−0.282	−0.18	0.244
n-butyrate	0.301	0.082	0.221	−0.171	−0.056	**.355***	−0.23	0.053	0.092	0.196	−0.207
i-valerate	−0.070	−0.026	−0.116	−0.279	−0.05	−0.012	−0.085	−0.065	−0.231	−0.015	0.090
n-valerate	0.228	0.153	0.130	−0.191	−0.075	0.040	−0.158	0.039	−0.161	−0.161	0.048

[1]*Bifidobacterium catenulatum/psudocatenulatum*, *$p<0.05$, **$p<0.01$

Table 7.
sIgA, short chain fatty acids and some bacteria showing significant correlation.

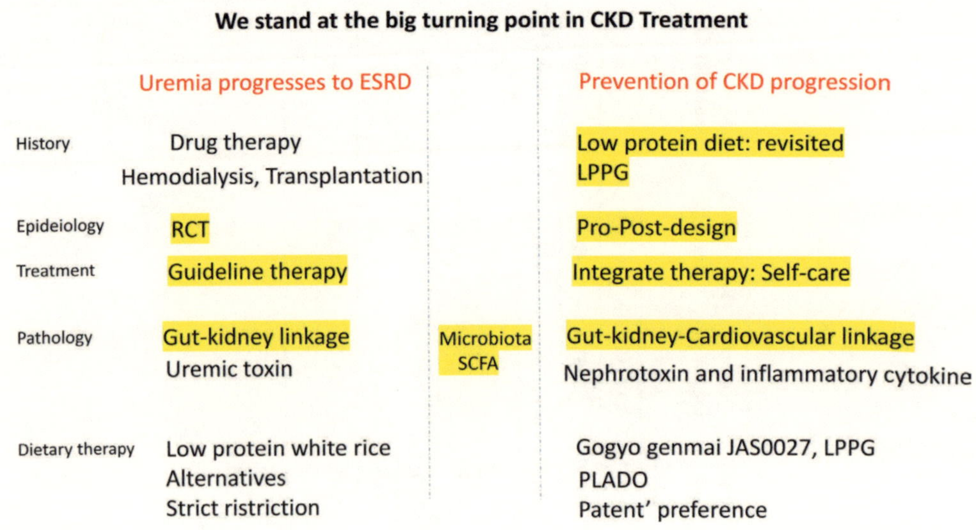

Figure 5.
Past and future direction of CKD treatment. Self care and integrated support becomes essential.

vegetables, binds phosphorus to phytate for insoluble absorption inhibition, reduces glomerular hyperfiltration with plant-based protein, and increases magnesium intake, among other benefits [5, 44–47]. LPPG satisfies all the above requirements.

Nakao et al. indicated that a low-protein diet is effective even in dialysis patients [57].

Additionally, the low phosphorus content of LPPG may reduce low FGF23-clotho gene products, which regulate phosphorus metabolism, potentially contributing to improved prognosis [58–60].

Some have expressed concerns that a low-protein diet may increase the risk of frailty or sarcopenia, but this is likely influenced by protein-energy malnutrition caused by low-energy diets in CKD rather than the reduction in protein intake itself.

Adopting a dietary therapy is essential in renal failure, but adherence is challenging. The number of dialysis patients remains high despite the development of drug therapy [61]. In regions with a rice-based diet, replacing white rice with LPPG alone allows for greater freedom in choosing tasty side dishes while maintaining good compliance with protein intake restrictions.

7. Conclusion

High-protein diets result in faster CKD progression and higher cardiovascular disease risk [62]. A fiber-rich low-protein diet with remaining functional ingredients of genmai and antioxidant activity leads to favorable alterations in the gut microbiome, which can modulate uremic toxin generation and slow CKD progression. LPPG is a heart-healthy, safe, flexible, and feasible diet that could be the centerpiece of a conservative and preservative CKD-management strategy that challenges the prevailing dialysis-centered paradigm [63].

Such dietary therapy requires the patient's independent action, especially when healthcare providers lack understanding of low-protein diets, it is necessary to approach it with the mindset of taking responsibility for one's health.

Author details

Shaw Watanabe[1]*, Shu Wakino[2], Yasushi Saiga[3], Katsuhiko Fukuda[4], Jun Mochizuki[5], Tan Wei[6], Qi Guo[7] and Haerani Rasyid[8]

1 Medical Rice Association and Tokyo University of Agriculture, Tokyo, Japan

2 Tokushima University, Tokushima, Japan

3 Hemodialysis Center, Fujii Hospital, Kishiwada, Japan

4 Shimane Integrative Medicine Clinic, Shimane, Japan

5 Technosuruga Lab, Shizuoka, Japan

6 Nanjing Medical University, Nanjing, China

7 Shanghai Chronic Disease Rehabilitation Research Center, China

8 Universitas Hasanuddin, Indonesia

*Address all correspondence to: gwatashaw@gmail.com

IntechOpen

© 2025 The Author(s). Licensee IntechOpen. This chapter is distributed under the terms of the Creative Commons Attribution License (http://creativecommons.org/licenses/by/4.0), which permits unrestricted use, distribution, and reproduction in any medium, provided the original work is properly cited.

References

[1] Polenakovic MH, Dohcev S, Rambabova-Bushljetik I, Gjorgjievski D, Spasovski G. The importance of the world kidney day world kidney day - 11 March 2021 - Living well with kidney disease. 2021;**42**(1):19-40. DOI: 10.2478/prilozi-2021-0002

[2] Watanabe S, Adachi K, Wakino S, al. Dietary therapy with low protein genmai to improve the gut-kidney axis and reduce CKD progression. Asia Pacific. The Journal of Clinical Nutrition. 2022;**31**:341-347

[3] Watanabe S. A trap of RCT in low protein dietary therapy. Reevaluation of pro-post study for dietary intervention. AS. Nutrition and Health. 2023;7:35-38

[4] Kistler BM, Moore D, Benner BA, Boaz M, et al. The International Society of Renal Nutrition and Metabolism Commentary on the National Kidney Foundation and academy of nutrition and dietetics KDOQI clinical practice guideline for nutrition in chronic kidney disease. Journal of Renal Nutrition. 2021;**31**(2):116-120.e1. DOI: 10.1053/j.jrn.2020.05.002

[5] Levin A, Ahmed SB, Carrero JJ, Foster B, Francis A, et al. Executive summary of the KDIGO 2024 clinical practice guideline for the evaluation and Management of Chronic Kidney Disease: Known knowns and known unknowns. Kidney International. 2024;**105**(4):684-701. DOI: 10.1016/j.kint.2023.10.016

[6] Hendricks AR. Practical topics and updates in renal pathology. Seminars in Diagnostic Pathology. 2020;**37**(3):115. DOI: 10.1053/j.semdp.2020.03.006

[7] Roberts I. Pathology of IgA nephropathy. Nature Reviews. Nephrology. 2014;**10**:445-454. DOI: 10.1038/nrneph.2014.92

[8] Marín R, Gorostidi M, Fernández-Vega F, Alvarez-Navascués R. Systemic and glomerular hypertension and progression of chronic renal disease: The dilemma of nephrosclerosis. Kidney International. Supplement. 2005;**99**:S52-S56. DOI: 10.1111/j.1523-1755.2005.09910.x

[9] The Wikimedia Foundation. Kobayashi Red Yeast Rice Scandal from Wikipedia. 2025. Available from: https://en.wikipedia.org/wiki/Kobayashi_red_yeast_rice_scandal

[10] Barbier O, Jacquillet G, Tauc M, Cougnon M, Poujeol P. Effect of heavy metals on, and handling by the kidney. Nephron. Physiology. 2005;**99**(4):105-110. DOI: 10.1159/000083981

[11] Lim YJ, Sidor NA, Tonial NC, Che A, Urquhart BL. Uremic toxins in the progression of chronic kidney disease and cardiovascular disease: Mechanisms and therapeutic targets. Toxins (Basel). 2021;**13**(2):142. DOI: 10.3390/toxins13020142

[12] Cai J, Chen Z, Wu W, Lin Q, Liang Y. High animal protein diet and gut microbiota in human health. Critical Reviews in Food Science and Nutrition. 2022;**62**(22):6225-6237. DOI: 10.1080/10408398.2021.1898336

[13] D'Apolito M, Du X, Pisanelli D, Pettoello-Mantovani M, Campanozzi A, et al. Urea-induced ROS cause endothelial dysfunction in chronic renal failure. Atherosclerosis. 2015;**239**:393-400

[14] Mihai S, Codrici E, Popescu I, et al. Inflammation-related mechanisms

in chronic kidney disease prediction, progression, and outcome. Journal of Immunology Research. 2018;**2018**:1-16

[15] Ashby D, Borman N, Burton J, Corbett R, Davenport A, et al. Renal association clinical practice guideline on Haemodialysis. BMC Nephrology. 2019;**20**(1):379. DOI: 10.1186/s12882-019-1527-3

[16] Pletinck A, Schepers E, Glorieux G. Biochemical and clinical impact of organic uremic retention solutes: A comprehensive update. Toxins. 2018;**10**:33

[17] Vaziri ND, Wong J, Pahl M, Piceno YM, Yuan J, et al. Chronic kidney disease alters intestinal microbial flora. Kidney International. 2013;**83**(2):308-315. DOI: 10.1038/ki.2012.345. Epub 2012 Sep 19

[18] Hobby GP, Karaduta O, Dusio GF, Singh M, Zybailov BL, Arthur JM. Chronic kidney disease and the gut microbiome. American Journal of Physiology. Renal Physiology. 2019;**316**(6):F1211-F1217. DOI: 10.1152/ajprenal.00298.2018. Epub 2019 Mar 13

[19] Cigarran Guldris S, González Parra E, Cases AA. Gut microbiota in chronic kidney disease. Nefrología. 2017;**37**(1):9-19. DOI: 10.1016/j.nefroe.2017.01.017

[20] Rysz J, Franczyk B, Ławiński J, Olszewski R, Ciałkowska-Rysz A, Gluba-Brzózka A. The impact of CKD on uremic toxins and gut microbiota. Toxins (Basel). 2021;**13**(4):252. DOI: 10.3390/toxins13040252

[21] Hirakawa A, Aoe S, Watanabe S, Hisada T, Mochizuki J, Mizuno S, et al. The nested study on the intestinal microbiota in GENKI study with special reference to the effect of brown rice eating. Journal of Obesity and Chronic Diseases. 2019;**3**:1-13

[22] Kikuchi K, Watanabe S, Matsuo M, et al. Changes in microbiota and short-chain fatty acids following 3-month pilot intervention study feeding Brown Rice ball (Omusubi) to healthy volunteers. Prensa Médica Argentina. 2021;**107**(2):315. DOI: 10.47275/0032-745X-315.38

[23] Imai E, Yasuda Y, Matsuo S. A decade after the KDOQI CKD guidelines: A perspective from Japan. American Journal of Kidney Diseases. 2012;**60**(5):729-730. DOI: 10.1053/j.ajkd.2012.08.025

[24] de Boer IH, Khunti K, Sadusky T, Tuttle KR, Neumiller JJ, Rhee CM, et al. Diabetes management in chronic kidney disease: A consensus report by the American Diabetes Association (ADA) and kidney disease: Improving global outcomes (KDIGO). Kidney International. 2022;**102**(5):974-989. DOI: 10.1016/j.kint.2022.08.012

[25] Goda T et al. Conceptualizing treatment strategies for diabetic kidney disease: The importance of early diagnosis and treatment. Juntendo Medical Journal. 2024;**70**(6):408-415

[26] Girardi ACC, Polidoro JZ, Castro PC, Pio-Abreu A, Noronha IL, Drager LF. Mechanisms of heart failure and chronic kidney disease protection by SGLT2 inhibitors in nondiabetic conditions. American Journal of Physiology. Cell Physiology. 2024;**327**(3):C525-C544. DOI: 10.1152/ajpcell.00143.2024

[27] Walker H, Khan S, Padmanabhan S, Pell JP, Lewsey J, et al. Analysis of the kidney failure risk equation implementation in routine clinical practice and health inequalities in chronic kidney disease care: A

retrospective cohort study. BMC Nephrology. 2025;**26**(1):113. DOI: 10.1186/s12882-025-04043-0

[28] Watanabe S. The potential health benefits of brown rice. In: Huang M, editor. Sustainable Rice Production-Challenges, Strategies and Opportunities. London, UK: IntechOpen; 2023. DOI: 10.5772/intechopen.104284

[29] Watanabe S, Takahashi M, Hashimoto H, Kikuchi K, Matsuo M. Medical rice; a new whole grain functional food for health and diseases. In: Functional Foods and Neutraceuticals in Metabolic and Non-communicable Diseases. London: Elsevier; 2020

[30] Takei N, Watanabe N, Nakajo M. Low-protein Rice (LPR) product: Processing method and product safety. Advances in Food Technology and Nutritional Sciences - Open Journal. 2017;**3**:33-41

[31] Jiang J, Xiong Y. Natural antioxidants as food and feed additives to promote health benefits and quality of meat products: A review. Meat Science. 2016;**120**:107-117

[32] Melekoglu E, Samur FG. Dietary strategies for gut-derived protein bound uremic toxins and cardio-metabolic risk factors in chronic kidney disease. A focus on dietary fibers. Critical Reviews in Food Science and Nutrition. 2021;**63**:3994-4008. DOI: 10.1080/10408398.2021.1996331

[33] Nagata N, Miyoshi-Akiyama T. Population-level metagenomics uncovers distinct effects of multiple medications on the human gut microbiome. Gastroenterology. 2022;**163**:1038-1052

[34] Takahashi M, Watanabe S, Mizuno S, Hirakawa A. Dietary and life habits of obesity and brown rice eaters among Genmai evidence for nutritional Kenko innovation (GENKI)study I and II. Clinical and Functional Nutrition. 2018;**10**(2):79-86

[35] Watanabe S. The founders of nutritional science (13) Sagen Ishizuka, 1851-1909. Clinical and Functional Nutriology. 2011;**3**(2):61

[36] Watanabe S, Mizuno S, Hirakawa A. Effects of brown rice on obesity: GENKI study I (cross sectional epidemiological study). Journal of Obesity and Chronic Diseases. 2018;**2**:12-19

[37] Watanabe S. Evaluation of three-color food guide. Clinical and Functional Nutriology. 2010;**2**(3):162-164

[38] GDB Chronic Kidney Disease Collaboration. Global, regional, and national burden of chronic kidney disease, 1990-2017:A systematic analysis for the global burden of disease study 017. Lancet. 2020;**395**(10225):709-733

[39] Watanabe S, Kashiwara N. The international conference on dietary therapy for chronic kidney disease with special reference to the gut-kidney linkage and low protein Brown Rice (Genmai). Diabetes Complications. 2023;**7**(1):1-3

[40] Levy AS, Greene T, Beck GJ, et al. Dietary protein restriction and the progression of chronic renal disease: What have all of the results of the MDRD study shown? Modification of diet in renal disease study group. Journal of the American Society of Nephrology. 1999;**10**:2426-2439

[41] Watanabe S, Adachi K, Iseki K. Prevention of diabetic nephropathy by low protein processed genmai Brown Rice. Diabetes Complications. 2024;**8**:1-5

[42] Yamamoto S, Watanabe S, For the JPHC Study Group. Geographic characteristics and mortality profiles in the JPHC study. Japan public health center-based prospective study on cancer and cardiovascular diseases. Journal of Epidemiology. 2001;**11**(6 Suppl):S8-S23

[43] Koppe L, Mafra D, Fouque D, et al. Probiotics and chronic kidney disease. Kidney International. 2015;**88**:958-966

[44] Zoccali C, Vanholder R, Massy ZA, Ortiz A, Sarafidis P, et al. The systemic nature of CKD. Nature Reviews Nephrology. 2017;**13**(6):344-358. DOI: 10.1038/nrneph.2017.52

[45] Cuspisti A et al. Plant-based diets in the management of CKD. American Journal of Kidney Diseases. 2007;**49**(6):962-973. DOI: 10.1053/j.ajkd.2007.03.003

[46] Wallace TC, Bailey RL, Blumberg JB, Burton-Freeman B, Chen CO, et al. Fruits, vegetables, and health: A comprehensive narrative, umbrella review of the science and recommendations for enhanced public policy to improve intake. Critical Reviews in Food Science and Nutrition. 2020;**60**(13):2174-2211. DOI: 10.1080/10408398.2019.16322 58

[47] Lee CC, Fan H, Tsopmo A, Regenstein JM, Ashaolu TJ. Plant-based antioxidant peptides: Impact on oxidative stress and gut microbiota. Critical Reviews in Food Science and Nutrition. Published online April 12, 2025. DOI: 10.1080/10408398.2025.24902 70

[48] Mizuno S, Watanabe S, Iseki K, et al. Proteinuria is a key factor predicting the progression of CKD: Nine-year follow-up of retrospective health examinee's cohort, Okinawa Study. Diabetes Complication. 2024;**8**(3):1-7

[49] Recharla N, Geesala R, Shi XZ. Gut microbial metabolite butyrate and its therapeutic role in inflammatory bowel disease: A literature review. Nutrients. 2023;**15**(10):2275. DOI: 10.3390/nu15102275

[50] Louis P, Flint HJ. Formation of propionate and butyrate by the human colonic microbiota. Environmental Microbiology. 2017;**19**(1):29-41. DOI: 10.1111/1462-2920.13589

[51] Maiuolo J, Bulotta RM, Ruga S, Nucera S, Macrì R, et al. The postbiotic properties of butyrate in the modulation of the gut microbiota: The potential of its combination with polyphenols and dietary fibers. International Journal of Molecular Sciences. 2024;**25**(13):6971. DOI: 10.3390/ijms25136971

[52] Miller BM, Liou MJ, Lee JY, Bäumler AJ. The longitudinal and cross-sectional heterogeneity of the intestinal microbiota. Current Opinion in Microbiology. 2021;**63**:221-230. DOI: 10.1016/j.mib.2021.08.004

[53] Li X, Hu S, Yin J, Peng X, King L, et al. Effect of symbiotic supplementation on immune parameters and gut microbiota in healthy adults: A double-blind randomized controlled trial. Gut Microbes. 2023;**15**(2):2247025. DOI: 10.1080/19490976.2023.2247025

[54] Schlosser P, Surapaneni AL, Borisov O, Schmidt IM, Zhou L, et al. Chronic renal insufficiency cohort (CRIC) study investigators and the CKD biomarkers consortium. Association of integrated proteomic and metabolomic modules with risk of kidney disease progression. Journal of the American Society of Nephrology. 2024;**35**(7):923-935. DOI: 10.1681/ASN.0000000000000343.44

[55] Nakao T, Kanazawa Y, Takahashi T. Once weekly hemodialysis combined with low-protein and low-salt dietary treatment as a favorable therapeutic modality for selected patients with end-stage renal failure: A prospective observational study in Japanese patients. BMC Nephrology. 2018;**19**:151-161

[56] Watanabe S, Ohtsubo K. Low-protein diet: History and use of processed low-protein rice for the treatment of chronic kidney disease. Foods. hypothesis. Toxins (Basel). 2022;**14**:221 2021:10:2255. DOI: 10.3390/foods 10102255

[57] Isakova T, Ix JH, Sprague SM, Raphael KL, Fried L, et al. Rationale and approaches to phosphate and fibroblast growth factor 23 reduction in CKD. Journal of the American Society of Nephrology. 2015;**26**(10):2328-2339. DOI: 10.1681/ASN.2015020117

[58] Stohr R, Schuh A, Heine G, Brandenburg V. FGF23 in cardiovascular disease: Innocent bystander or active mediator? Frontiers in Endocrinology. 2018;**9**:351

[59] Russo D, Battaglia Y. Clinical significance of FGF-23 in patients with CKD. International Journal of Nephrology. 2011;**2011**:1-5

[60] Scialla J, Appel L, Wolf M, et al. Plant protein intake is associated with fibroblast growth factor 23 and serum bicarbonate levels in patients with chronic kidney disease: The chronic renal insufficiency cohort study. Journal of Renal Nutrition. 2012;**22**:379-388.e1

[61] Japan Hemodialysys Association. Current Report of Chronic Dialysis in Japan. 2023. Available from: https://docs.jsdt.or.jp/overview/file/2023/pdf/02.pdf

[62] Levin A et al. The effects of a low-protein, plant-based diet on kidney function in patients with CKD: A randomized controlled trial. American Journal of Kidney Diseases. 2019;**73**(4):495-503. DOI: 10.1053/j.ajkd.2018.09.023

[63] Rhee CM, Wang AY-M, Biruete A, Kistler B, Kovesdy CP, Zarantonell D, et al. Nutritional and dietary management of chronic kidney disease under conservative and preservative kidney care without dialysis. Journal of Renal Nutrition. 2023;**33**:S56-S66. DOI: 10.1053/j.jrn.2023.06.010

Chapter 4

Metabolic Syndrome and Its Effects on the Reno-Vascular System

Nivedha Balaji, Crystal Ayazo and Idopise Umana

Abstract

Metabolic syndrome is a constellation of interconnected conditions such as hypertension, insulin resistance, diabetes mellitus, and dyslipidemia that contribute to atherosclerotic vascular disease, leading to myocardial infarction, cerebrovascular accidents, and peripheral arterial disease. Metabolic syndrome propagates renovascular injury, ultimately leading to chronic kidney disease. The global prevalence of metabolic syndrome is up to 39%, and its incidence continues to rise. The syndrome exerts multifactorial effects on renal pathophysiology, including cytokine release and oxidative stress that drive systemic inflammation, mitochondrial dysfunction, and activation of the renin-angiotensin-aldosterone system. Insulin resistance contributes to hyperfiltration, glomerulosclerosis, and microvascular remodeling resulting in macromolecular leakage and renal disease. Furthermore, conditions such as hyperuricemia and metabolic dysfunction-associated fatty liver disease further deterioration of renal function. Therefore, it is essential to understand the pathomechanisms underlying metabolic syndrome-associated kidney disease and develop strategies to prevent or delay the progression of renal dysfunction.

Keywords: metabolic syndrome, renovascular disease, chronic kidney disease, hypertension, hyperglycemia, insulin resistance, hyperlipidemia, hypertriglyceridemia, dyslipidemia, obesity, chronic inflammation

1. Introduction

Metabolic syndrome (MetS) is a constellation of various metabolic derangements including visceral adiposity/central obesity, insulin resistance/hyperglycemia, hypertension (HTN), and atherogenic hyperlipidemia/dyslipidemia that can raise one's risk for developing atherosclerotic cardiovascular disease, type 2 diabetes, nonalcoholic fatty liver disease, myocardial infarction, stroke, and chronic kidney disease (CKD) [1–6]. MetS is defined as having at least 3 of the following characteristics - an elevated waist circumference with population-defined specifications, elevated triglycerides ≥150 mg/dl, reduced high-density lipoprotein (HDL) <40 mg/dl in males or < 50 mg/dl in females, elevated systolic blood pressure ≥ 130 mmHg or elevated diastolic pressure ≥ 85 mmHg, elevated fasting glucose ≥100 mg/dl [7, 8].

This multifactorial condition affects up to 39% of people worldwide [9]. One-fifth of the American and European populations and one-fourth of the Latin American population are reported to have MetS [2]. According to the National Health and

Nutrition Examination Survey in 2009–2010, there was a MetS prevalence of 22% and 24% in females and males, respectively [10]. Systematic reviews and meta-analyses have shown that prevalence varies by region, with rates of 12% in rural populations and 22.5% in urban populations [9]. Although the disease is commonly seen among adults, with an incidence of 40% in individuals over the age of 60, the multifactorial condition has also been reported among children. The incidence of MetS was noted in 3% of children and 5% of adolescents in 2020 [2].

With the rising incidence of MetS, there is an increase in MetS-associated chronic diseases directly impacting healthcare costs. In the United States alone, annual healthcare expenditures attributable to MetS have exceeded half a trillion dollars, with additional indirect costs linked to lost productivity and workforce impact [1, 4]. Additionally, there is an increase in morbidity and excess premature mortality [4].

Currently, there is a vast amount of research on the implications of MetS and the development of cardiovascular diseases such as myocardial infarction and stroke; however, studies have shown that there is a 1.4-to-4.4-fold increase in developing chronic kidney disease [4]. Therefore, there is a need for a detailed understanding of the associations between the mechanisms of MetS and chronic renal disease. The chapter will focus on the pathogenesis of MetS and elucidate how to prevent or delay the progression of renal dysfunction.

2. The mechanisms of MetS-related renovascular disease

CKD is a debilitating disease characterized by the persistence of an estimated glomerular filtration rate of <60 mL/min/1.73 m^2, urinary albumin to creatinine ratio ≥ 30 mg/g, or albuminuria ≥30 mg per day for at least 3 months [11, 12]. CKD is a global epidemic with a prevalence of 14% worldwide. In 2016, an estimated 26 million individuals were living with CKD in the United States [11]. MetS-related kidney disease presents as glomerulopathy, podocytopathy, mesangial and matrix proliferation, tubular atrophy, interstitial fibrosis, glomerular basement membrane, and global, and segmental sclerosis. The pathomechanisms of MetS-Related CKD are multifactorial and complex, including insulin resistance, adiposity, hypertension, inflammation, oxidative stress, and hyperuricemia. This section will review the mechanisms of renovascular injury present in Metabolic Syndrome.

2.1 Insulin resistance, hyperglycemia, inflammatory stress

Diabetic kidney disease is a multifaceted impairment of the renal vascular system secondary to hyperglycemia-mediated dysregulation of intracellular metabolism, inflammation, increased apoptosis, and tissue fibrosis. Diabetic nephropathy presents with glomerular hypertrophy resulting in hyperfiltration, glomerular and tubulointerstitial inflammation, and disordered cellular apoptosis [13].

Glomerular hyperfiltration is meditated by the growth hormone/insulin-like growth factor (IGF-1) system. 40–50% of the protein makeup of IGF-1 is identical to that of the insulin molecule. Afferent arteriole dilatation mediated by IGF-1, prostaglandins, bradykinin, nitric oxide, and atrial natriuretic peptide along with thromboxane A2 mediated efferent arteriole constriction results in glomerular hyperfiltration [14]. Hyperinsulinemia results in the overactivation of the Akt signaling pathway which upregulates endothelial nitric oxide synthase in the vascular and renal tissue [8]. The abundance of endothelial nitric oxide synthase resulting in a surplus of nitric oxide contributes to glomerular hyperfiltration [14]. The excess nitric oxide causes vasorelaxation, leukocyte and monocyte adhesion to the renal vasculature, activates platelet aggregation, and induces proinflammatory cytokines [8].

Additionally, hyperinsulinemia increases endothelin-1 production, a potent vasoconstrictor that exacerbates microvascular endothelial dysfunction and increases glomerular capillary permeability, resulting in albuminuria [3, 15]. Insulin resistance also contributes to podocyte loss and glomerular basement membrane (GBM) disruption, promoting proteinuria and progressive renal failure [5].

Additionally, the hyperglycemia-induced release of chemokines like ornithine decarboxylase causes increased filtration and renal hypertrophy. Hyperglycemia also results in sodium-glucose co-transporters 2 (SGLT2) upregulation within the proximal convoluted tubules. This causes maximal reabsorption within the proximal convoluted tubules, thereby increasing glomerular filtration and triggering activation of the renin-angiotensin-aldosterone system (RAAS). RAAS is activated due to low sodium delivered to the distal tubules [16].

Metabolically derived derangements in MetS cause subsequent inflammation termed "metainflammation" [3]. Both hyperglycemia and adiposity activate the proinflammatory pathways via cytokines, chemokines, adipokines, and oxidative stress [3, 5].

Insulin resistance results in insufficient glycemic control leading to the production of advanced glycation end-products (AGEs) that potentiate inflammatory signaling pathways, induce oxidative stress, and exacerbate vascular injury resulting in renal damage [8, 17]. AGEs synthesize nuclear factor κB (NF-κB) and reactive oxygen species (ROS) which initiate cellular growth or hypertrophy, inflammation, angiogenesis, endovascular dysfunction, and extracellular matrix deposition [18].

Hyperglycemia causes activation of protein kinase C (PKC) in the renal cortex. This triggers an abnormal activation of cellular signaling pathways and gene expression. It also increases endothelial permeability and synthesis of extracellular matrix proteins that propagate vascular dysfunction [17]. PKC also stimulates NF-κB which releases interleukin-6 and tumor necrosis factor-α (TNF-α) by endothelial and mesangial cells. Both AGE and PKC activate downstream pro-oxidative pathways [13].

The polyol pathway metabolizes excess glucose into sorbitol which causes osmotic damage and oxidative stress resulting in renal injury and dysfunction [17]. The hexosamine pathway produces proteoglycans, glycolipids, and glycoproteins. Glutamine: fructose-6-phosphate-amidotransferase (GFAT) is an essential enzyme in this pathway. Glomerular cells in humans lack this rate-limiting enzyme; however, in hyperglycemic environments, there is an overexpression of GFAT which stimulates TGF-β1 production. Furthermore, PKC potentiates this process resulting in increased inflammation [18]. Insulin resistance shifts the glycolytic pathway towards the polyol and hexosamine pathways resulting in oxidative stress and NF-κB mediated inflammation [16].

Animal studies have shown that elevated oxidized low-density lipoprotein and E-selectins recruit pro-inflammatory macrophages to the kidneys [3]. Adipocytokines release from adipocytes stimulate macrophage chemoattractant protein-1 (MCP-1), macrophage migration inhibitory factor, chemokine ligand 5, and macrophage colony-stimulating factor which results in glomerulosclerosis and widespread fibrosis causing proteinuria and renal dysfunction. Additionally, this stimulates ROS in the kidneys that alter renal tubular transportation, induces TGF-β1, triggers nuclear factor-κ mediated fibrinolysis, and increases nicotinamide adenine dinucleotide phosphate oxidase (NADPH) pathways within the B cells. Furthermore, an overexpression of zymogen activator inhibitor 1 aggravates renal fibrosis [5].

Also, there is a rise in leptin seen with both excessive adiposity and hyperinsulinemia which promotes the secretion of angiotensin II and aldosterone, which enhances the secretion of plasminogen activator inhibitor-1 and TGF-β1 [8, 14]. This activates the mineralocorticoid receptors which are overexpressed in adipose tissue. The consequential proinflammatory environment and oxidative stress induce vascular remodeling and atherosclerosis. This increases type IV collagen deposition causing renal tubular atrophy, interstitial fibrosis, and glomerulosclerosis. Additionally, there is an increase in sodium reabsorption via the RAAS [5, 8].

Obesity also activates aldosterone-independent ligands such as Ras-related C3 botulinum toxin substrate 1, reactive oxygen species, and activated 11β-hydroxysteroid dehydrogenase 1, increasing cortisol levels. Subsequently, there is an increase in mineralocorticoid receptor activation in the renal tubules causing an elevation of blood pressure [8]. Resistin, an adipose sensor, also contributes to obesity, albuminuria, and progression of kidney disease. Some studies have shown that resistin enhances the expression of intracellular adhesion molecule-1 and vascular cell adhesion molecule-1 which upregulate the sympathetic nervous system in the kidneys [3].

Hyperinsulinemia also induces renal tubular lipid deposition. Insulinemia increases TGF-β1 from adipocytes which propagates lipid accumulation in the tubular cells causing tubular atrophy and interstitial fibrosis. The abundance of TGF-β1 leads to increased activity of sterol regulatory element binding protein-1 [5, 8]. Hyperinsulinemia also induces the production of IGF-1, which stimulates connective tissue growth factor (CTGF). CTCF has pro-fibrogenic effects on renal tubular and interstitial fibrosis. IGF-1 also decreases matrix metalloproteinase-2 activity, which is involved in extracellular matrix degradation. Thus, there is increased extracellular matrix expansion in addition to renal fibrosis [14].

Visceral adiposity and renal fat deposition via cytokines such as TNF-α and IL-6 induce neovascularization. MetS-driven microvascular proliferation is mediated by the overexpression of vascular endothelial growth factor (VEGF) due to hyperinsulinemia and dyslipidemia. Initially, the upregulated microvascularization contributes to renal perfusion accounting for an elevated renal blood flow and glomerular filtration rate. Subsequently, due to the disorganized architecture of the microvessels, they become more tortuous and unstable. Thus, leading to dysfunctional intra-renal and glomerular capillaries. Furthermore, in the setting of glomerular hyperfiltration, there is an increased risk of microvascular loss and progression of renal disease [3].

Furthermore, with co-existing hyperglycemia secondary to insulin resistance in MetS, there is an increased anti-naturetic effect. Insulin causes increased sodium reabsorption, thereby increasing the blood pressure. With increased glomerular pressures, there is a hypertrophic effect on the proximal epithelial cells causing further elevation in arterial pressures [3].

2.2 Hypertension and the renin-angiotensin-aldosterone system (RAAS)

HTN, defined as a systolic blood pressure ≥ 130 mmHg or diastolic pressure ≥ 85 mmHg is a key component of MetS [7, 8]. Obesity is thought to be the major contributor that links HTN to MetS. The RAAS plays a critical role in blood pressure regulation by modulating vasculature tone and fluid status through renal salt absorption [1, 3, 15]. Angiotensin II in the RAAS binds to vascular smooth muscle receptors in the proximal tubular cells resulting in sodium resorption and efferent arteriole vasoconstriction with afferent arteriole vasodilation which causes increased vascular osmolality and expansion resulting in elevated blood pressure. Additionally, angiotensin II increases sodium reabsorption in the distal nephron via aldosterone binding to the mineralocorticoid receptors. This leads to an increase in blood pressure [8, 15].

Visceral adipocytes in MetS store and secrete increased levels of angiotensin II and angiotensinogen precursors along with aldosterone resulting in excessive activation of the RAAS system [1, 15, 19]. Animal studies have shown that after 1 week of high-fat diet consumption, blood pressure rises by 6% [20]. Angiotensin II and Aldosterone in the RAAS induce fibrotic activity in the reno-vascular endothelium and proximal tubular cells [3]. Excessive stimulation of the RAAS leads to higher renal volume burden and hyperfiltration. Thus, damaging and disrupting the glomerular filtration barrier, including the endothelium, basement membrane, and podocytes [5].

Additionally, increased adiposity causes cardiac and renal baroreceptor dysfunction resulting in the overactivity of the sympathetic nervous system. Adipose tissue triggers the central proopiomelanocortin pathway, especially in sleep apnea and obesity causing carotid body chemoreceptor stimulation thus raising the blood pressure [1, 8]. Obesity increases leptin and reduces adiponectin which triggers the sympathetic nervous system and increases aldosterone levels contributing to HTN [3, 5]. Leptin released from fat cells releases α-melanocyte-stimulating hormones that bind to the melanocortin-4 receptors in the hypothalamus, brainstem, and spinal cord that stimulate the sympathetic nervous system [8]. This rise in sympathetic activity triggers a release of catecholamines, prostaglandins, and renin that elevate blood pressure [1, 15].

Excess visceral and retroperitoneal fat in central obesity increases intra-abdominal pressure that compresses the kidneys. This accelerates the development of HTN. Excess intra-abdominal pressure compresses the thin loop of Henle and the vasa recta of the renal medulla. This decreases the tubular flow rate and sodium excretion. The macula densa is then stimulated by renin secreted by juxtaglomerular cells. The RAAS is activated to increase renal blood flow and glomerular filtration. This potentiates the RAAS resulting in a self-perpetuating cycle [3, 8].

The long-term effect of elevated systemic vascular HTN is increased glomerular pressures. This results in renal damage and ischemia. Furthermore, the ischemia induces angiotensin II synthesis and secretion in an effort to increase renal perfusion that potentiates renovascular constriction and renal parenchymal proliferation damaging the kidneys [5].

2.3 Obesity

Excess adiposity has been strongly associated with an increased risk of chronic kidney disease. The pathomechanisms are mostly attributed to insulin resistance and elevated blood pressure [19]. The effects of obesity-related hyperinsulinemia and hypertension have been mentioned in previous sections.

Hormone dysregulation and abnormal adiposity modify renal structure and function termed Obesity-related glomerulopathy [5]. With increased adiposity and weight, each podocyte undergoes a mechanical stretch to accommodate the increase in glomerular volume. This results in decreased podocyte density and increased foot process width. Animal studies show that, initially, there is an equivocal growth in podocyte size and glomerular hypertrophy. However, gradually, podocyte growth slows down compared to the extent of glomerular hypertrophy. The podocytes subsequently detach resulting in glomerular basement membrane denudation. This results in segmental sclerosis, which potentiates macromolecular leakage and proteinuria. This is known as obesity-related glomerulopathy [3, 5]. Obesity-related glomerulopathy has increased 10-fold in the last 15 years [14].

Approximately 12% of individuals with obesity-related glomerulopathy can progress to focal segmental glomerulosclerosis [3]. Additionally, the excess lipid molecules found in innate renal cells including the podocytes lead to renal cell energy depletion [5]. The excess perirenal lipids within the renal sinus promote oxidative stress and proinflammatory cytokines through the cytotoxic effects of intracellular triglycerides. The increase in triglycerides causes a toxic accumulation of toxic metabolites, such as ceramides, that potentiate intrinsic renal cell apoptosis resulting in CKD [5, 8]. Studies have shown that stages of CKD can be correlated to plasma ceramide levels independent of other risk factors. An accumulation of perirenal fat within the renal sinus also causes endoplasmic reticulum stress due to oxidative stress and inflammation. This results in mitochondrial dysfunction and cellular apoptosis [8].

2.4 Oxidative stress and mitochondrial dysfunction

Oxidative stress produces reactive oxygen species that damage proteins, lipids, and deoxyribonucleic acid. Oxidative stress plays a pivotal role in the development of MetS [3, 14].

Oxidative stress upregulates nicotinamide adenine dinucleotide phosphate oxidase (NOX) enzymes which stimulate ROS production in the renal glomeruli. The upregulation of ROS damages podocytes, endothelial cells, and mesangial cells potentiating CKD. In mouse models, hyperglycemia results in augmented NOX activity and subsequent ROS which causes cellular apoptosis and podocyte loss [3]. Furthermore, an inappropriate activation of the NOX enzyme results in pancreatic β-cell and liver damage that causes glucolipotoxicity. This promotes the progression of MetS to diabetes [14].

Lipid peroxidation which is the breakdown of fatty acids in lipid membranes by free radicals correlates with body mass index and waist circumference [3]. Lipid peroxidation generates low-density lipoproteins (LDL) that accumulate in the renal mesangial cells generating foam cells. This can trigger an inflammatory response that activates macrophages, impairs vasodilatory action, and damages the endothelium. Lipid peroxidation stimulates the generation of more ROS and free radicals augmenting further kidney damage [14].

Mitochondrial ROS-mediated glomerular hyperfiltration is another cause of renal damage in MetS. Oxidative stress results in an overproduction of prostaglandin E2 and overactivation of cyclooxygenase-2 gene transcription. This activates the nuclear factor-κB pathway. This results in an increase in angiotensin II. Additionally, oxidative stress augments the release of Angiotensin II. Angiotensin II then propagates a vicious cycle of mitochondrial ROS production. The effects of angiotensin II on blood pressure and glomerular fibrosis have been described earlier. In MetS, the surplus of nutrients augments the electron supply to the respiratory chain. However, due to the low demand for adenosine triphosphate, from immobility and lack of physical activity, there is a disproportionate number of superoxides formed. This potentiates mitochondrial dysfunction [14].

Oxidized LDL impairs oxidation–reduction reactions across the mitochondrial membrane and translocates mitochondrial proteins leading to vascular endothelial dysfunction and apoptosis. NOX-derived ROS disrupts the electron transport chain, impairs mitochondrial function, and deposits extracellular matrix protein in mesangial cells [14]. The expansion of mesangium and accumulation of cellular debris within the matrix forms Kimmelstiel and Wilson nodules [16]. In MetS, the AMPK pathway is inactivated. The AMPK pathway protects cells by regulating PPAR-γ coactivator-1α in a calorie-deprived state and inhibits the mammalian target of rapamycin, which is involved in NOX-induced podocyte dysfunction. This pathway inactivates the mitochondrial production of ROS. Moreover, mitochondrial malfunction has been associated with the development of type 2 diabetes mellitus. Studies have shown that a 35% reduction in mitochondrial DNA has been seen in peripheral blood cells preceding the diagnosis of type 2 diabetes. These studies describe the vital role of mitochondrial function in modulating energy metabolism and developing MetS-related renal complications [14].

2.5 Hyperuricemia

Hyperuricemia is characterized by an elevated serum uric acid, greater than greater than 7.0 mg/dL in men and 6.0 mg/dL in women. The overproduction or underexcretion of uric acid during purine metabolism is hyperuricemia. While classically linked to gout, recent evidence suggests a broader systemic role in metabolic syndrome and cardiovascular diseases [21]. Individuals with uric acid levels <6 mg/dL have a 5.9% prevalence of Mets while the prevalence increases to 59% in individuals with uric acid levels at 10 mg/dL or greater [3].

MetS—characterized by central obesity, insulin resistance, dyslipidemia, and hypertension—frequently coincides with hyperuricemia. Elevated serum uric acid is considered a possible early marker and pathogenic factor for MetS. Uric acid may impair insulin signaling and promote oxidative stress and endothelial dysfunction, aggravating the metabolic profile [3, 21, 22]. On the other hand, fructose intake, commonly elevated in MetS, increases uric acid synthesis. Uric acid, in turn, stimulates hepatic fat accumulation and impairs nitric oxide bioavailability, creating a vicious cycle contributing to both insulin resistance and hypertension [22]. Additionally, uric acid also inhibits nitric oxide production resulting in the inability to accomplish vasodilation. This increases glomerular capillary wall vulnerability and permeability, resulting in albuminuria [3].

In the kidneys, hyperuricemia contributes to renovascular disease by promoting vascular smooth muscle proliferation, increasing systemic and glomerular pressure, and inducing inflammation. This results in preglomerular arteriolopathy and cortical ischemia—pathophysiological hallmarks of uric acid-induced kidney injury [22].

In experimental models, uric acid activates the renin-angiotensin system, exacerbates oxidative stress, and induces macrophage infiltration in renal tissues. These changes precede overt renal dysfunction, suggesting a mechanistic role in early renovascular damage, particularly in individuals with MetS [22].

2.6 Metabolic dysfunction-associated fatty liver disease

Metabolic dysfunction-associated fatty liver disease (MAFLD) is characterized by increased fat deposition in the liver in the absence of significant alcohol intake or other secondary causes of steatohepatitis. However, it occurs in the presence of metabolic risk factors such as obesity, hypertension, insulin resistance, and dyslipidemia. Studies have shown that patients with MetS have up to 3.7-fold higher incidence of MAFLD [8]. There is a bidirectional relationship between insulin resistance and dyslipidemia seen in MetS with MAFLD. Insulin resistance is thought to propagate lipotoxicity by causing lipid accumulation in hepatic tissue, causing downstream inflammation both within and outside the liver. This inflammatory process invokes cytokines such as TNF-α and IL-6, to further escalate the metabolic imbalance [23].

3. Prevention and management of MetS-related renovascular disease

Individuals with uncontrolled in comparison to controlled MetS are at a 3.28 times greater risk for developing rapid decline in kidney function. Therefore, early recognition and treatment of MetS is pivotal in preventing and delaying the progression of reno-vascular disease. This section will discuss lifestyle changes and management of hyperglycemia, hypertension, hyperlipidemia, and hyperuricemia.

3.1 Lifestyle modifications

Lifestyle interventions in individuals with MetS include dietary modifications, physical activity, avoidance of tobacco products, reduced alcohol consumption, reduced caffeine consumption, and good sleep hygiene. People should aim for a goal of up to 10% body weight reduction over 1 year or a target body mass index of less than 25 kg/m^2. The American Heart Association and American College of Cardiology recommend a weekly goal of 150 minutes of moderate-intensity activity or 70 minutes of high-intensity activity. Additionally, diets should be abundant in fruits, vegetables, whole grains, legumes, and nuts while minimal in processed foods, refined carbohydrates, saturated fats, and increased sodium [2].

3.2 Weight loss

Weight loss improves both inflammatory (TNF-α, IL-6, leptin) and anti-inflammatory (adiponectin) markers involved in MetS-associated nephropathy. A previous study has shown that a 5% reduction in weight in obese women can reduce RAAS activity in adipose tissue and plasma [3].

In addition to diet modification and increased physical activity, anti-obesity medications may also be considered. Sympathomimetics that suppress appetite include phentermine and diethylpropion. However, these medications are associated with elevated heart rate, elevated blood pressure, insomnia, constipation, and dry mouth. These medications are contraindicated in people with uncontrolled hypertension, underlying cardiovascular disease, hyperthyroidism, and glaucoma. Orlistat is an intestinal lipase inhibitor that can reduce up to 30% of lipid absorption. Topiramate is a carbonic-anhydrase inhibitor that promotes taste aversion and reduces caloric intake. Buproprion-naltrexone combines a dopamine and norepinephrine reuptake inhibitor with a μ-opioid receptor antagonist that decreases cravings and appetite. This is associated with nausea, vomiting, constipation, headache, dry mouth, dizziness, and insomnia [24].

Glucagon-like peptide-1 such as liraglutide and semaglutide decreases appetite and increases satiety. These medications are contraindicated in individuals with a personal or familial history of medullary thyroid cancer or multiple endocrine neoplasia type 2. Tirzepatide is a dual glucagon-like peptide-1 and glucose-dependent insulinotropic peptide receptor agonist. It reduces caloric intake, increases insulin sensitivity, and increases glucose and triglyceride uptake in adipose tissue. The SURMOUNT trials noted that tirzepatide was associated with significant weight loss, improved glycemic control, and improved cardiometabolic risk factors (waist circumference, blood pressure, and cholesterol). SYNERGY-NASH, a phase 2 study, noted that a greater proportion of individuals achieved resolution of metabolic-associated steatohepatitis without worsening liver fibrosis in a patient treated with tirzepatide when compared to the placebo group after 52 weeks of treatment [24].

Setmelanotide is a melanocortin-4-receptor agonist that decreases appetite. It is indicated in people with monogenic obesity secondary to pro-opiomelanocortin, proprotein convertase subtilisin/kexin type 1, or leptin receptor deficiency. This is commonly associated with hyperpigmentation. Gelesis100 is a hydrogel matrix composed of modified cellulose structures and citric acid to achieve satiety by increasing water absorption. This can be associated with bloating, infrequent bowel movements, or dyspepsia [24].

Other off-label medications are associated with weight loss. Bupropion is a norepinephrine and dopamine reuptake inhibitor that is associated with a small weight loss when compared to other antidepressants, which usually cause weight gain. Metformin suppresses gluconeogenesis and increases peripheral insulin sensitivity. Weight loss with metformin is linked to increased leptin sensitivity, increased activation of AMPK, and increased anorexigenic hormones. Pramlintide mimics pancreatic amylin, which mediates postprandial blood sugar. Sodium-glucose transport-2 (SLGT-2) inhibitors promote glucosuria by reducing the renal threshold for glucose reabsorption. Several studies, including the EMPAREG CVOT, have shown that SGLT-2 inhibitors are associated with weight loss. However, they increase one's risk for urinary tract infections, genital mycotic infections, and dehydration [24].

Bariatric surgery is an alternative effective means of weight loss that reduces the long-term risk of progression of kidney dysfunction [8]. Surgical procedures such as laparoscopic banding, Roux-en-Y gastric bypass, or laparoscopic sleeve gastrectomy are recommended for patients with BMI $\geq$ 40 kg/m^2 or BMI $\geq$ 35 kg/m^2 and other comorbidities [2]. While bariatric surgery has peri and postoperative risks such as infections, respiratory failure, renal failure, increased mortality, and complications such as malabsorption or nephrolithiasis, trials have shown that surgery can significantly reduce blood pressure and blood glucose, even resulting in diabetes regression [8]. A previous study among adolescents showed an average estimated glomerular filtration rate rise of 26 ml/min/1.73 m^2 3 years post-bariatric surgery. A six-year follow-up study in patients post gastric bypass surgery showed that the risk of kidney disease progression was reduced by 45% [5].

3.3 Antihypertensive therapy

Hypertension is a defining component of metabolic syndrome and a leading contributor to the development and progression of renovascular damage. According to the 2017 ACC/AHA hypertension guidelines, pharmacologic therapy in patients with blood pressure greater than 130/80 mmHg is recommended in patients with a formal diagnosis of type 2 diabetes mellitus, CKD, or established cardiovascular disease [25]. In patients with MetS-related renovascular disease, blood pressure management is essential not only to reduce cardiovascular risk but also to prevent progression to ischemic nephropathy.

ACE inhibitors and ARBs are considered first-line agents, particularly in proteinuria or diabetes. These agents reduce intraglomerular pressure and proteinuria and have been shown to slow the progression of renal disease with added cardiovascular benefits [26]. However, caution is required in patients with bilateral renal artery stenosis or a solitary kidney, as these drugs can precipitate rapid declines in glomerular filtration and hence cause acute kidney injury [27].

The CORAL trial demonstrated that optimal medical therapy, which included ACE inhibitors, calcium channel blockers, diuretics, and statins, was as effective as renal artery stenting in reducing cardiovascular and renal events in patients with atherosclerotic renal artery stenosis. The study emphasized that interventional procedures should be reserved for refractory cases and that pharmacologic therapy is effective in most patients with stable disease [28]. Additional reviews have reinforced the importance of renin-angiotensin system blockade (ACE inhibitors and ARBs) in mitigating proteinuria and preserving renal function, even in patients with significant renal artery stenosis [26, 27]. Clinical practice should include close monitoring of serum creatinine and potassium following initiation to detect any acute kidney injury.

Moreover, renal denervation (RDN), though novel, has become an increasingly well-established intervention for patients with uncontrolled hypertension, particularly those with MetS. By attenuating renal sympathetic nerve activity, RDN offers significant blood pressure reduction. This is crucial for slowing the progression of renovascular damage commonly seen in MetS [29]. In addition to its antihypertensive effects, RDN may improve insulin sensitivity and modulate systemic inflammation. This contributes to vascular injury and atherogenesis in MetS-related renovascular disease [30]. Therefore, RDN represents a promising adjunct in the prevention and management of renovascular complications.

Ultimately, initial therapy with ACE inhibitors or ARBs is recommended, particularly in the presence of proteinuria or diabetes [25]. If further blood pressure control is needed, calcium channel blockers or thiazide-like diuretics can be added. Regular monitoring and patient-specific risk stratification are necessary to guide the safe and effective use of these agents in MetS-related renovascular disease [27, 28].

3.4 Antilipidemic therapy

Dyslipidemia, particularly elevated triglycerides and low HDL-C is a hallmark of MetS and a major driver of atherosclerotic changes in renal arteries. The 2018 ACC/AHA cholesterol guidelines advocate for high-intensity statin therapy in adults with diabetes or clinical ASCVD, conditions often overlapping with MetS-related renovascular disease [31].

Statins reduce LDL-C, improve endothelial function, and have anti-inflammatory properties that contribute to vascular protection [32]. Patients with MetS often have lipid abnormalities, including elevated triglycerides and low HDL-C that drive vascular inflammation and endothelial dysfunction. Statins not only lowered LDL-C but also reduced vascular inflammation, oxidative stress, and plaque instability, all of which are implicated in the progression of renal artery stenosis and parenchymal ischemia [32, 33].

The SHARP trial provided robust evidence that simvastatin and ezetimibe when combined significantly reduced major atherosclerotic events in patients with chronic kidney disease, regardless of baseline lipid levels [34]. Although MetS patients were not specifically isolated, the pathophysiology overlaps substantially, reinforcing the benefit of lipid-lowering in this population. Additionally, a comprehensive review by Bragança noted that statins in MetS reduce oxidative stress and vascular stiffness, which are key contributors to renovascular remodeling. Moreover, lipid abnormalities in MetS may contribute to renal lipotoxicity, an emerging contributor to kidney injury and fibrosis. These findings support early initiation of statin therapy in patients with renovascular disease and metabolic syndrome [33].

Moreover, high-intensity statins, such as atorvastatin or rosuvastatin, are recommended in MetS patients with renovascular involvement [31]. Ezetimibe may be added for additional LDL-C reduction or in cases of statin intolerance. In patients with familial hypercholesterolemia or extremely high ASCVD risk, PCSK9 inhibitors may be considered for additional benefit [31, 34]. Lifestyle interventions remain foundational but insufficient when used without pharmacologic therapy in high-risk individuals [32, 33].

3.5 Antiglycemic therapy

Insulin resistance and hyperglycemia are central to the MetS and exacerbate renovascular damage through endothelial dysfunction, increased RAAS activation, and chronic inflammation. The ADA guidelines advocate for a target HbA1c <7% in most non-pregnant adults, with an emphasis on early initiation of agents that provide cardiovascular and renal protection, such as SGLT2 inhibitors and GLP-1 receptor agonists [35]. These medications have been shown to improve renal outcomes beyond glycemic control due to their ability to lower glomerular pressure, reduce tubular workload, and modulate inflammatory pathways. Their effects are crucial in MetS, where insulin resistance and low-grade inflammation perpetuate renal and vascular damage [36].

The EMPA-REG OUTCOME trial conducted in patients with type 2 diabetes and cardiovascular disease demonstrated a significant reduction in cardiovascular deaths and slowed kidney disease progression when treated with empagliflozin. These findings are relevant for patients with MetS and renovascular disease due to the shared pathophysiological mechanisms involved [37]. Similarly, the CREDENCE trial confirmed renal and cardiovascular protection with canagliflozin by reducing the risk of end-stage kidney disease and renal death in patients with diabetic nephropathy.

Furthermore, a review by Alicic emphasized that in MetS, where hyperglycemia and hyperinsulinemia drive both glomerular hypertension and arterial inflammation, SGLT2 inhibitors reduce renal injury independently of HbA1c. GLP-1 receptor agonists also attenuate inflammatory and atherogenic processes that worsen renovascular disease [35].

Metformin remains first-line for type 2 diabetes in MetS unless contraindicated due to advanced kidney disease or gastrointestinal intolerance. SGLT2 inhibitors should be initiated early on in patients with renovascular diseases or elevated risk for cardiovascular diseases [37]. GLP-1 receptor agonists such as liraglutide and semaglutide should be added for additional weight loss or cardiovascular protection. Insulin or sulfonylureas have not shown significant renal benefit. Additionally, these medications have adverse side effects such as weight gain and hypoglycemia [35, 36].

3.6 Hyperuricemia management

Targeting uric acid may offer therapeutic benefits in MetS and chronic kidney disease (CKD). Xanthine oxidase inhibitors like allopurinol and febuxostat reduce uric acid production and improve endothelial function. Emerging agents, such as dotinurad—a selective URAT1 inhibitor—show promise in enhancing uric acid excretion and mitigating renal injury without increasing cardiovascular risk [21].

Early intervention in hyperuricemic individuals with MetS may delay CKD progression and reduce cardiovascular events. However, more randomized controlled trials are needed to establish causality and determine optimal uric acid targets.

Hyperuricemia is a modifiable risk factor with growing recognition as a contributor to the pathogenesis of metabolic syndrome and renovascular disease. Its role extends beyond crystal deposition to include systemic effects that impact insulin sensitivity, vascular function, and renal integrity. Addressing hyperuricemia may represent a promising strategy in the integrated management of cardio-renal-metabolic disorders.

4. Conclusions

Metabolic syndrome is a multifaceted disorder composed of the interplay between insulin resistance, hypertension, increased adiposity, pro-inflammatory pathways, and oxidative stress. There is a growing global burden of metabolic syndrome-related complications, including chronic kidney disease. Early screening with primary care providers emphasizing lifestyle and dietary changes to prevent the development of metabolic syndrome should be practiced. Upon the development of chronic kidney disease, nephrologists should initiate management to minimize disease progression. Future studies should emphasize cost-effective therapies that mitigate patient mortality and morbidity.

Funding

Our chapter did not receive any funding source.

Conflict of interest

The authors declare no conflict of interest.

Author details

Nivedha Balaji*, Crystal Ayazo and Idopise Umana
Northeast Georgia Medical Center, Gainesville, Georgia, USA

*Address all correspondence to: niveb95@outlook.com

IntechOpen

© 2025 The Author(s). Licensee IntechOpen. This chapter is distributed under the terms of the Creative Commons Attribution License (http://creativecommons.org/licenses/by/4.0), which permits unrestricted use, distribution, and reproduction in any medium, provided the original work is properly cited.

References

[1] Soleimani M, Barone S, Luo H, Zahedi K. Pathogenesis of hypertension in metabolic syndrome: The role of fructose and salt. International Journal of Molecular Sciences. 2023;**24**:4294. DOI: 10.3390/ijms24054294

[2] Swarup S, Ahmed I, Grigorova Y, et al. Metabolic syndrome. In: StatPearls [Internet]. Treasure Island (FL): StatPearls Publishing; 2025. Available from: https://www.ncbi.nlm.nih.gov/books/NBK459248/ [Accessed: March 7, 2024]

[3] Zhang X, Lerman LO. The metabolic syndrome and chronic kidney disease. Translational Research. 2017;**183**:14-25. DOI: 10.1016/j.trsl.2016.12.004

[4] Ndumele CE, Rangaswami J, Chow SL, Neeland IJ, Tuttle KR, Khan SS, et al. Cardiovascular-kidney-metabolic health: A presidential advisory from the American Heart Association. Circulation. 2023;**148**(20):1606-1635. DOI: 10.1161/CIR.0000000000001184

[5] Lin L, Tan W, Pan X, Tian E, Wu Z, Yang J. Metabolic syndrome-related kidney injury: A review and update. Frontiers in Endocrinology. 2022;**13**:904001. DOI: 10.3389/fendo.2022.904001

[6] Spahis S, Borys JM, Levy E. Metabolic syndrome as a multifaceted risk factor for oxidative stress. Antioxidants & Redox Signaling. 2017;**26**(9):445-461. DOI: 10.1089/ars.2016.6756

[7] Saklayen MG. The global epidemic of the metabolic syndrome. Current Hypertension Reports. 2018;**20**(2):12. DOI: 10.1007/s11906-018-0812-z

[8] Scurt FG, Ganz MJ, Herzog C, Bose K, Mertens PR, Chatzikyrkou C. Association of metabolic syndrome and chronic kidney disease. Obesity Reviews. 2024;**25**(1):e13649. DOI: 10.1111/obr.13649

[9] Zila-Velasque JP, Grados-Espinoza P, Challapa-Mamani MR, Sánchez-Alcántara F, Cedillo-Balcázar J, Cs AD, et al. Prevalence of metabolic syndrome and its components according to altitude levels: A systematic review and meta-analysis. Scientific Reports. 2024;**14**(1):27581. DOI: 10.1038/s41598-024-77928-z

[10] Lovre D, Mauvais-Jarvis F. Trends in prevalence of the metabolic syndrome. Journal of the American Medical Association. 2015;**314**(9):950. DOI: 10.1001/jama.2015.8625

[11] Vaidya SR, Aeddula NR. Chronic kidney disease. In: StatPearls [Internet]. Treasure Island (FL): StatPearls Publishing; 2025. Available from: https://www.ncbi.nlm.nih.gov/books/NBK535404/ [Accessed: July 31, 2024]

[12] Thomas MC, Brownlee M, Susztak K, Sharma K, Jandeleit-Dahm KA, Zoungas S, et al. Diabetic kidney disease. Nature Reviews. Disease Primers. 2015;**1**:15018. DOI: 10.1038/nrdp.2015.18

[13] Gembillo G, Ingrasciotta Y, Crisafulli S, Luxi N, Siligato R, Santoro D, et al. Kidney disease in diabetic patients: From pathophysiology to pharmacological aspects with a focus on therapeutic inertia. International Journal of Molecular Sciences. 2021;**22**(9):4824. DOI: 10.3390/ijms22094824

[14] Ruan X, Guan Y. Metabolic syndrome and chronic kidney disease. Journal of Diabetes. 2009;**1**(4):236-245. DOI: 10.1111/j.1753-0407.2009.00042.x

[15] De Bhailis ÁM, Kalra PA. Hypertension and the kidneys. British Journal of Hospital Medicine (London, England). 2022;**83**(5):1-11. DOI: 10.12968/hmed.2021.0440

[16] Qazi M, Sawaf H, Ismail J, Qazi H, Vachharajani T. Pathophysiology of diabetic kidney disease. EMJ Nephrology eJournals. 2022;**10**(1):102-113. DOI: 10.33590/emjnephrol/22-00060

[17] Kumar M, Dev S, Khalid MU, Siddenthi SM, Noman M, John C, et al. The bidirectional link between diabetes and kidney disease: Mechanisms and management. Cureus. 2023;**15**(9):e45615. DOI: 10.7759/cureus.45615

[18] Agarwal R. Pathogenesis of diabetic nephropathy. In: Chronic Kidney Disease and Type 2 Diabetes. Arlington (VA): American Diabetes Association; 2021. Available from: https://www.ncbi.nlm.nih.gov/books/NBK571720/doi:10.2337/db20211-2

[19] Zhu D, Judge PK, Wanner C, Haynes R, Herrington WG. The prevention and management of chronic kidney disease among patients with metabolic syndrome. Kidney International. 2025;**107**(5):816-824. DOI: 10.1016/j.kint.2024.12.021

[20] Armitage JA, Burke SL, Prior LJ, Barzel B, Eikelis N, Lim K, et al. Rapid onset of renal sympathetic nerve activation in rabbits fed a high-fat diet. Hypertension. 2012;**60**(1):163-171. DOI: 10.1161/HYPERTENSIONAHA.111.190413

[21] Yanai H, Adachi H, Hakoshima M, Katsuyama H. Molecular biological and clinical understanding of the pathophysiology and treatments of hyperuricemia and its association with metabolic syndrome, cardiovascular diseases and chronic kidney disease. International Journal of Molecular Sciences. 26 Aug 2021;**22**(17):9221. DOI: 10.3390/ijms22179221. PMID: 34502127; PMCID: PMC8431537

[22] Johnson RJ, Nakagawa T, Jalal D, Sanchez-Lozada LG, Kang DH, Ritz E. Uric acid and chronic kidney disease: Which is chasing which? Nephrology, Dialysis, Transplantation. 2013;**28**(9):2221-2228. DOI: 10.1093/ndt/gft029

[23] Cariou B, Byrne CD, Loomba R, Sanyal AJ. Nonalcoholic fatty liver disease as a metabolic disease in humans: A literature review. Diabetes, Obesity & Metabolism. 2021;**23**(5):1069-1083. DOI: 10.1111/dom.14322

[24] Tchang BG, Aras M, Kumar RB, et al. Pharmacologic treatment of overweight and obesity in adults. In: Feingold KR, Ahmed SF, Anawalt B, et al., editors. Endotext [Internet]. South Dartmouth (MA): MDText.com, Inc.; 2000. Available from: https://www.ncbi.nlm.nih.gov/books/NBK279038/ [Accessed: August 20, 2024]

[25] Whelton PK, Carey RM, Aronow WS, et al. 2017 ACC/AHA/AAPA/ABC/ACPM/AGS/APhA/ASH/ASPC/NMA/PCNA guideline for the prevention, detection, evaluation, and management of high blood pressure in adults. Circulation. 2018;**138**(17):e484-e594. DOI: 10.1161/CIR.0000000000000596

[26] Cooper CJ, Murphy TP, Cutlip DE, Jamerson K, Henrich W, Reid DM, et al. CORAL Investigators. Stenting and medical therapy for atherosclerotic renal-artery stenosis. The New England Journal of Medicine. 2 Jan 2014;**370**(1):13-22. DOI: 10.1056/NEJMoa1310753. Epub 2013 Nov 18. PMID: 24245566; PMCID: PMC4815927

[27] Safian RD, Textor SC. Renal-artery stenosis. The New England Journal of Medicine. 2001;**344**(6):431-442. DOI: 10.1056/NEJM200102083440607

[28] Cooper CJ, Murphy TP, Cutlip DE, et al. Stenting and medical therapy for atherosclerotic renal-artery stenosis. The New England Journal of Medicine. 2014;**370**(1):13-22. DOI: 10.1056/NEJMoa1310753

[29] Mahfoud F, Schmieder RE, Azizi M, Pathak A, Sievert H, Tsioufis C, et al. Proceedings from the 2nd European Clinical Consensus Conference for device-based therapies for hypertension: State of the art and considerations for the future. European Heart Journal. 21 Nov 2017;**38**(44):3272-3281. DOI: 10.1093/eurheartj/ehx215. Erratum in: European Heart Journal. 1 May 2018;**39**(17):1534. DOI: 10.1093/eurheartj/ehx290. PMID: 28475773; PMCID: PMC5837218

[30] Verloop WL, Spiering W, Vink EE, Beeftink MM, Blankestijn PJ, Doevendans PA, et al. Denervation of the renal arteries in metabolic syndrome: The DREAMS-study. Hypertension. Apr 2015;**65**(4):751-757. DOI: 10.1161/HYPERTENSIONAHA.114.04798. Epub 2015 Feb 2. PMID: 25646297

[31] Grundy SM, Stone NJ, Bailey AL, et al. 2018 AHA/ACC/multi-society guideline on the management of blood cholesterol. Journal of the American College of Cardiology. 2019;**73**(24):e285-e350. DOI: 10.1016/j.jacc.2018.11.003

[32] Ginsberg HN. Insulin resistance and cardiovascular disease. The Journal of Clinical Investigation. 2000;**106**(4):453-458. DOI: 10.1172/JCI10762

[33] Sharp Collaborative Group. Study of Heart and Renal Protection (SHARP): Randomized trial to assess the effects of lowering low-density lipoprotein cholesterol among 9,438 patients with chronic kidney disease. American Heart Journal. Nov 2010;**160**(5):785-794.e10. DOI: 10.1016/j.ahj.2010.08.012. Epub 2010 Sep 18. PMID: 21095263

[34] Baigent C, Landray MJ, Reith C, et al. The effects of lowering LDL cholesterol with simvastatin plus ezetimibe in patients with chronic kidney disease (SHARP): A randomized placebo-controlled trial. Lancet. 2011;**377**(9784):2181-2192. DOI: 10.1016/S0140-6736(11)60739-3

[35] Alicic RZ, Rooney MT, Tuttle KR. Diabetic kidney disease: Challenges, progress, and possibilities. Clinical Journal of the American Society of Nephrology. 2017;**12**(12):2032-2045. DOI: 10.2215/CJN.11491116

[36] Gheith O, Farouk N, Nampoory N, Halim MA, Al-Otaibi T. Diabetic kidney disease: Worldwide difference of prevalence and risk factors. Journal of Nephropharmacology. 2016;**5**(1):49-56

[37] Zinman B, Wanner C, Lachin JM, et al. Empagliflozin, cardiovascular outcomes, and mortality in type 2 diabetes. The New England Journal of Medicine. 2015;**373**(22):2117-2128. DOI: 10.1056/NEJMoa1504720

Chapter 5

Updates on Calcific Uremic Arteriolopathy: Impact, Diagnosis, and Treatment

Wen Wen

Abstract

Calcific uremic arteriolopathy (CUA), or calciphylaxis, is a rare but life-threatening disorder predominantly affecting patients with end-stage renal disease. Characterized by painful ischemic skin lesions and a high mortality rate, CUA's pathogenesis involves mineral metabolic imbalances, vascular smooth muscle cell osteogenic transformation, microthrombosis, inflammation, and genetic susceptibility. Diagnosis remains challenging due to the variability of clinical presentation and overlapping skin disorders; thus, a combination of clinical assessment, biopsy, and imaging is recommended. Current management protocols are multidisciplinary, focusing on correcting metabolic derangements, optimizing dialysis, aggressive wound care, and multimodal pain control. Therapies such as sodium thiosulfate, cinacalcet, SNF472, and vitamin K supplementation are being explored, while interventions like surgical debridement and hyperbaric oxygen therapy may be beneficial for selected patients. Despite ongoing therapeutic advances, prognosis remains poor, and further research is needed to clarify underlying mechanisms and develop targeted treatment strategies.

Keywords: calcific, calciphylaxis, renal failure, pain, vitamin K, dialysis, thrombosis

1. Introduction

Calcific uremic arteriolopathy (CUA), commonly referred to as calciphylaxis, is a rare and life-threatening syndrome that predominantly affects individuals with chronic kidney disease (CKD), with the highest prevalence observed in patients with end-stage renal disease (ESRD) undergoing dialysis. Current reports indicate that CUA occurs in approximately 1–4% of patients receiving hemodialysis [1, 2]. Additional risk factors include Caucasian ethnicity, female sex, obesity, diabetes mellitus, elevated parathyroid hormone levels, and the use of vitamin K antagonists (e.g., warfarin), vitamin D supplements, or calcium phosphate binders [3]. Clinically, CUA is characterized by painful ischemic skin lesions, tissue necrosis, and an alarmingly high mortality rate, presenting formidable challenges in pathogenesis, diagnosis, and clinical management.

Despite decades of investigation, the underlying mechanisms of CUA remain incompletely understood, and current clinical approaches are often complex and, at times, unsatisfactory. The rising incidence and lethal complexity of CUA in at-risk populations underscore the urgent need for deeper insight into its molecular triggers and systemic imbalances. This chapter provides a thorough review of recent advances in understanding the pathogenesis, diagnosis, and treatment of CUA, highlighting critical knowledge gaps and proposing directions for future research.

2. Pathogenic mechanisms in CUA

CUA is not merely a passive consequence of vascular calcium deposition; rather, it is an active and multifaceted process that closely resembles osteogenesis, characterized by medial vascular calcification, intimal fibrosis, and thrombosis. A pivotal event in this pathology is the transdifferentiation of vascular smooth muscle cells (VSMCs) into osteoblast-like cells—a process known as osteogenic transdifferentiation. This transformation is orchestrated by a convergence of mineral metabolic imbalances, upregulation of osteogenic signaling pathways, loss of endogenous calcification inhibitors, and adverse microenvironmental factors such as inflammation and oxidative stress [4]. Collectively, these influences reprogram vascular cells to acquire bone-forming properties, ultimately resulting in pathological calcification.

In the following sections, we will examine the mechanisms driving CUA by focusing on four key aspects:

2.1 Mineral imbalance

Abnormalities in mineral metabolism, particularly elevated serum calcium and phosphate levels, have been strongly implicated in the pathogenesis of CUA [5]. The prevailing hypothesis posits that an increased calcium-phosphate product promotes the ectopic deposition of calcium-phosphate-apatite crystals within the vasculature of susceptible individuals. Nevertheless, several clinical studies have demonstrated that a significant proportion of patients with CUA may exhibit normal serum concentrations of calcium, phosphate, and parathyroid hormone (PTH) [6]; thus, challenging the notion that mineral imbalance alone is sufficient to precipitate the condition.

Furthermore, observations reveal that some patients experience an elevated risk of calciphylaxis following parathyroidectomy [7]—a procedure that precipitates an abrupt decrease in PTH and alters bone turnover dynamics. This phenomenon suggests that not only persistent hypermineralemia but also rapid shifts in bone metabolism and compensatory metabolic adaptations may contribute to the pathogenesis of CUA. The hypothesis that adynamic bone disease and the consequent impairment in buffering circulating calcium and phosphate predispose to vascular calcification continues to attract scholarly interest.

Many experts now propose that vascular calcification, including calciphylaxis, arises from a disturbance in the delicate balance between pro-calcific and anti-calcific factors (examples are listed in **Table 1**), rather than from mineral imbalance alone [8]. Key endogenous inhibitors of ectopic calcification—such as fetuin-A, matrix Gla protein (MGP), and pyrophosphate—are normally present in the circulation to prevent unregulated deposition of calcium-phosphate complexes. Notably, patients with end-stage renal disease, particularly those receiving dialysis, often display reduced circulating levels of these inhibitors. However, the precise mechanisms by which

Factors promoting calcification
Bone morphogenetic protein 2 (BMP-2)
Calcium-phosphate product
Tumor necrosis factor α (TNF-α)
Interleukin 6 (IL-6)
Receptor activator of nuclear factor κB (RANK) ligand (RANKL)
Insulin-like growth factor I (IGF-I)
Insulin
Glucose
Parathyroid hormone
Matrix metalloproteinases (MMP)
Elastin degradation
Hydroxyapatite crystals
Factors inhibiting calcification
Fetuin-A
Matrix gla protein (MGP)
Osteoprotegerin (OPG)

Table 1.
Pro-calcific and anti-calcific factors contributing to CUA.

a deficiency in these protective factors facilitates the development of CUA remain incompletely elucidated.

In addition, mounting evidence indicates that inflammation and oxidative stress play pivotal roles in promoting vascular calcification [9, 10]. Elevated levels of reactive oxygen species (ROS) and pro-inflammatory cytokines may induce endothelial dysfunction and stimulate the osteogenic transformation of vascular smooth muscle cells. Despite these insights, the exact cascade of events connecting systemic inflammation to focal cutaneous calcification is not fully defined. The intricate interplay between inflammation, systemic comorbidities—including diabetes, obesity, and autoimmune disorders—and local vascular changes underscores the need for further research to clarify whether inflammation acts as a primary instigator or as a secondary response within the calcification process.

2.2 Microthrombi and coagulation abnormalities

Microthrombus formation is a more distinguishing pathological feature of CUA than arteriole calcification itself, underscoring the importance of coagulation abnormalities in the disease process [11]. Recent clinical investigations have further clarified the critical roles of microthrombi formation and hemostatic dysregulation in the pathogenesis of CUA [12]. This multifaceted disorder arises from a complex interplay among vascular calcification, endothelial dysfunction, and disturbances in coagulation.

On the one hand, calcification of small arterioles—particularly within the medial layer—results in progressive vascular stenosis and chronic tissue ischemia. This chronic ischemia induces endothelial cell injury, creating a prothrombotic environment by promoting the release of tissue factor (TF) and adhesion molecules [13]. These mediators further activate platelets and the coagulation cascade. On the other hand, persistent endothelial injury disrupts the delicate balance between calcification inhibitors and promoters, as well as the local immunological milieu [14], thereby accelerating pathological calcium deposition within the vessel wall. In addition, endothelial dysfunction and pro-inflammatory cytokines—including interleukin-6 (IL-6) and tumor necrosis factor-alpha (TNF-α)—upregulate procoagulant factors such as von Willebrand factor while simultaneously downregulating endogenous anticoagulant pathways. Immune dysregulation, as seen in systemic conditions like lupus nephritis, can exacerbate activation of the coagulation cascade. A multicenter retrospective study redefines calciphylaxis as a subcutaneous, bone-forming microvascular injury syndrome chiefly mediated by complement pathway activation, particularly through C5b-9 deposition. The research highlights a strong association between complement-mediated endothelial injury, ensuing vascular thrombosis, and localized as well as systemic complement pathway activation, often in patients with uremic risk factors such as diabetes, obesity, and dialysis dependency [14].

Moreover, patients with CUA frequently display deficiencies in vitamin K-dependent anticoagulant proteins, notably protein C and protein S, which predispose them to a hypercoagulable state and subsequent microthrombosis [12]. Abnormal coagulation factors, such as elevated prothrombin fragments, further contribute to the high incidence of thrombus formation in small vessels, even in the absence of systemic hypercoagulability.

Vitamin K deficiency or antagonism—most notably due to warfarin therapy—impairs the γ-carboxylation of MGP, a crucial natural inhibitor of vascular calcification [15]. As a result, nonfunctional MGP fails to inhibit the deposition of calcium-phosphate complexes, thereby accelerating vascular calcification and promoting a prothrombotic microenvironment. Warfarin use in patients with end-stage renal disease (ESRD) has been shown to increase the risk of CUA by three- to thirteen-fold [16].

2.3 Genetic predisposition

Notably, despite the widespread prevalence of traditional risk factors—such as chronic kidney disease, diabetes, and obesity—among the dialysis population, only a small proportion of individuals develop CUA. This observation strongly suggests the involvement of genetic or other molecular predispositions. A study from the German Calciphylaxis Registry examined potential genetic risk factors for CUA in dialysis patients, with particular focus on polymorphisms in the genes encoding CD73 (NT5E), the vitamin D receptor, and fibroblast growth factor 23 (FGF23). Analysis of 165 single-nucleotide polymorphisms (SNPs) across 10 candidate genes revealed nominal, though not statistically robust, associations between specific SNPs within CD73, FGF23, and the vitamin D receptor genes and an increased risk of calciphylaxis [17]. The rarity of CUA within a broadly defined high-risk population further points to the likely contribution of as-yet-unidentified genomic elements or epigenetic modifications conferring susceptibility. To date, research in this area has been limited by small sample sizes and retrospective study designs, highlighting the need for larger, prospective studies to clarify the role of genetic polymorphisms and molecular markers in the pathogenesis of CUA.

3. Diagnostic progress and challenges

Early and accurate diagnosis of CUA is essential, given its high morbidity and mortality rates. However, the diagnostic process presents significant challenges. The reliance on clinical judgment is further complicated by considerable inter-patient variability. Some individuals with advanced CUA may initially manifest only subtle cutaneous changes, while others progress rapidly to widespread necrosis, resulting in potential diagnostic delays.

CUA typically presents as painful, ischemic skin lesions that may progress to necrotic ulcers, often covered by eschars. Although these characteristic findings are highly suggestive of CUA, they are not pathognomonic. Similar dermatologic manifestations can be observed in conditions such as cellulitis, venous stasis ulcers, and vasculitic disorders, necessitating careful clinical evaluation and thorough differential diagnoses (**Table 2**) [18]. Laboratory assessments, including measurements of serum calcium, phosphate, and parathyroid hormone (PTH), are routinely performed; however, their diagnostic utility for CUA is limited. Many patients with CUA exhibit laboratory values within normal ranges, particularly when metabolic changes are abrupt or compensated by other physiologic mechanisms. Additionally, while novel biomarkers such as circulating fetuin-A and matrix Gla protein have been proposed [19], their clinical validation is ongoing, and routine measurement has not yet been standardized.

Skin biopsy remains a cornerstone in the diagnosis of CUA. Histopathologically, CUA is characterized by medial calcification, intimal fibrosis, and microthrombosis of small arterioles in the dermis and subcutaneous tissue [5]. Nonetheless, several limitations exist: (1) sampling errors and sensitivity: In the early stages of CUA, calcifications may be focal or sparse, resulting in false-negative biopsy findings. Furthermore, technical factors such as insufficient tissue depth or suboptimal processing may compromise the detection of calcifications. (2) Risk of wound complications: Due to the impaired wound healing associated with CUA, skin biopsies can exacerbate local tissue injury, promote further calcification (koebnerization), and increase the risk of secondary infection. Studies have identified necrosis, finely stippled calcium, and intimal fibroplasia of pannicular arterioles as the most robust histopathologic features for diagnosing calciphylaxis, though inter-rater concordance for intimal fibroplasia remains low [11]. Quantitative analysis of pathologists' subjective assessments may further inform the development of diagnostic criteria and enhance medical education.

In recent years, various imaging modalities have been evaluated as adjunctive tools in the diagnosis of CUA. Plain radiographs and computed tomography (CT)

Warfarin-induced skin necrosis
Arterial atherosclerotic ischemic ulcer
Metastatic calcinosis cutis
Dystrophic calcinosis cutis
Monckeberg's arteriolosclerosis
Ulcer induced by venous stasis
Bacterial, mycotic, or parasitic cellulitis
Atheroembolism
Livedoid vasculopathy
Oxalosis
Pyoderma gangrenosum
Disseminated intravascular coagulation
Purpura fulminans
Systemic nephrogenic fibrosis

Table 2.
Differential diagnoses of CUA.

scans can demonstrate soft tissue calcifications, but these findings lack specificity for CUA. Nuclear medicine techniques, such as technetium-99 m bone scintigraphy, may reveal increased radionuclide uptake in areas of soft tissue calcification, providing supportive diagnostic evidence [20]. However, these methods can produce false-positive results in patients with diffuse vascular calcification unrelated to CUA.

The diagnosis of CUA remains challenging due to the inherent limitations of individual diagnostic modalities (**Table 3**). Integrated diagnostic strategies that combine clinical, histopathological, and imaging findings offer a more robust approach and are strongly warranted. Effective multidisciplinary collaboration among dermatologists, nephrologists, radiologists, and pathologists is essential for the accurate identification of CUA and for minimizing the risk of misdiagnosis, which can lead to delays in appropriate management. Diagnostic criteria are particularly valuable when histological confirmation is unavailable. For example, McCarthy et al. have proposed the Mayo criteria (**Table 4**), while Zhang et al. have introduced the Zhong Da criteria (**Table 5**).

Diagnostic method	Advantages	Limitations
Clinical examination	Immediate, noninvasive, cost-effective	Non-specific; similar findings in other conditions
Skin biopsy	Provides histological confirmation	Risks include poor wound healing and sampling errors
Radiographic imaging	Detects soft tissue calcifications	Low specificity; may not distinguish CUA from other calcifications
Nuclear bone scan	Highlights areas of abnormal uptake	Risk of false positives; limited accessibility
Ultrasound-guided core biopsy	Minimizes tissue trauma compared to open biopsy	Requires expertise; may still risk local complications

Table 3.
Comparison of diagnostic modalities in CUA.

	Clinical criteria[c]					
Skin biopsy criteria[b]	2 Major	1 Major	3 Minor	2 Minor	1 Minor	None
1 Major	Definite	Definite	Definite	Definite	Definite	Probable
2 Minor	Definite	Definite	Definite	Probable	Possible	Possible
1 Minor	Definite	Probable	Probable	Possible	Possible	No
ND or none[a]	Definite	Probable	Probable	Possible	No	No

[a]ND = not done.
[b]Skin biopsy criteria: Major = Medial calcification and intimal fibroplasia of panicular arterioles with cutaneous necrosis; Minor = Extravascular calcium deposition OR thrombosis of pannicular or dermal arterioles.
[c]Clinical criteria: Major = Necrotic cutaneous ulcers over indurated plaque OR Indurated plaque without ulcer in adipose-rich tissue including abdominal pannus, breasts, buttocks, and thighs; Minor = Livedo racemosa OR Hemorrhagic plaques OR Hemorrhagic bullae.

Table 4.
Mayo criteria [21].

Hierarchical diagnosis	Basis
Suspected diagnosis	a: There are 2 major factors, or 1 major factor and 3 minor factors.
	b: There are early suspicious skin changes, such as diffuse rash, purpura, subcutaneous induration, painful papules, cellulitis-like erythema and so on.
	c: Exclude other diseases that need to be identified
Clinical diagnosis	a: At least 1 risk factor is present.
	b: There are typical skin lesions, including livedo reticularis, painful purpura, painful or hemorrhagic violet plaques and indurations, necrotic ulcers and black eschar.
	c: Exclude other diseases that need to be identified
Confirmed diagnosis	a: Skin biopsy results are positive, showing calcification of subcutaneous microvessels, intimal fibrosis with microthrombosis, extravascular calcium deposition, and ischemic necrosis of epidermis, dermis and subcutaneous tissues.
	b: Presence of skin lesions: typical lesions or early suspicious changes
	c: Exclude other diseases that need to be identified

Risk factors: Major factors include dialysis over 5 years, long-term use of warfarin, use of high-dose calcium-phosphate binders exceeding 6 months, active vitamin D dose greater than 0.5 g/day, plasma protein C or protein S deficiency, vitamin K deficiency, and iPTH above 1000 pg./mL. And minor factors include dialysis less than 5 years, obesity, diabetes, hypoalbuminemia, long-term use of immunosuppressants and glucocorticoids, hypercalcemia, hyperphosphatemia, hyperalkaline phosphatasemia, iPTH below 300 pg./mL, subcutaneous injection of insulin or heparin, and iron overload.
Diseases that need to be identified: Including diabetic ulcer, atherosclerotic vascular disease, thromboangiitis obliterans, cellulitis, traumatic ulcer, dystrophic calcification, cholesterol embolism syndrome, vasculitis, pyoderma gangrenosum, stasis ulcer, neuropathic ulcer, warfarin-induced skin necrosis, nephrogenic systemic fibrosis and cryofibrinogenemia.

Table 5.
Zhong Da criteria [22].

4. Therapeutic challenges and emerging treatment strategies

Management of CUA is complicated by its multifactorial etiology, high morbidity, and the risk of treatment-associated complications. There is still no approved therapy for calciphylaxis; current treatment strategies are primarily supportive and aim at controlling pain, preventing infections, and correcting underlying metabolic imbalances. The mainstay of current CUA management includes optimal wound care, regulation of mineral metabolism, and strategies to regulate calcification and coagulation. There is interest in agents that specifically target the process of calcium-phosphate precipitation. Adjustments in the dialysis regimen, such as using a low-calcium bath and optimizing dialysis adequacy, have been proposed to mitigate hypercalcemia and minimize the risk of further calcification. Current guidelines recommend cinacalcet as first-line therapy for CUA in secondary hyperparathyroidism, given its targeted action on mineral metabolism dysregulation. Drugs such as sodium thiosulfate, bisphosphonates, and vitamin K supplements are being evaluated for their ability to modify the course of CUA by reducing calcific burden directly.

4.1 Inhibition of vascular calcification

4.1.1 Sodium thiosulfate (STS)

Sodium thiosulfate (STS) acts as detoxicant through the chelation of calcium ions, forming soluble calcium thiosulfate complexes. It also inhibits hydroxyapatite crystallization and exhibits both antioxidant and anti-inflammatory properties. A meta-analysis involving 358 patients demonstrated a 70.1% rate of lesion improvement and marked pain reduction following STS therapy, underscoring its dual role in mitigating pathological calcification and alleviating symptoms [23]. Retrospective cohort studies further substantiate these benefits, with 58% of patients (n = 52) achieving complete ulcer epithelialization within 6 months of treatment [5]. Established dosing regimens commonly involve intravenous administration of 25 g (100 mL of a 25% solution) three times per week, typically during the final 30–60 minutes of each hemodialysis session [24]. Notably, possibly due to ethnic differences, Chinese patients often exhibit reduced tolerance to the standard dose of STS. To address this, Zhang et al. have proposed an optimized regimen for Chinese patients, recommending a maximum dose of 10 g (250 mL of a 4% solution) per administration [25]. While topical application of STS has been utilized, its efficacy is likely limited by poor penetration to the deep lesions characteristic of CUA. Additionally, there are reports suggesting that intralesional (IL) STS (250 mg/mL) may effectively manage patients with localized cutaneous involvement [26].

Notably, comparative analyses indicate that STS confers a mortality reduction benefit superior to that of traditional phosphate binders, reflected by a hazard ratio (HR) of 0.62 for survival outcomes—an effect attributed to its calcium-chelating properties and multifaceted mechanisms targeting the underlying vascular pathology [21]. While meta-analyses from all the available cohort studies suggest that STS improves lesion outcomes, no statistically significant increase in overall survival has been observed [27]. Nevertheless, these findings position STS as a cornerstone in the therapeutic armamentarium for calciphylaxis, offering an effective balance between clinical efficacy and practical utility.

4.1.2 SNF472 (hexasodium fytate)

SNF472, a novel hexasodium salt of myoinositol hexaphosphate, exerts its therapeutic effect by selectively inhibiting hydroxyapatite crystallization. Its mechanism of action involves direct binding to calcium-phosphate complexes within soft tissues, thereby preventing pathological mineralization while preserving physiological bone calcification. The pivotal CALCIPHYX Phase III trial provides clinical validation [28]. Although the trial did not meet its primary endpoints—improvement in wound healing (BWAT-CUA scores) and pain (VAS)—it reduced calciphylaxis-related hospitalizations and deaths compared to placebo, suggesting the potential benefits in important clinical outcomes and warranting further research on its therapeutic role [29]. This targeted therapeutic profile positions SNF472 as a paradigm-shifting agent in the management of vascular calcification, addressing both the efficacy limitations and safety concerns associated with legacy therapies.

4.2 Thrombolysis and anticoagulation: Targeting microvascular occlusion

4.2.1 Tissue plasminogen activator (tPA)

The use of low-dose tPA was first mentioned by Sewell et al. [30]. Tissue plasminogen activator (tPA) exerts its thrombolytic effect by binding to fibrin within thrombi and catalyzing the conversion of plasminogen to plasmin—a serine protease that degrades fibrin strands, thereby dissolving occlusive clots. This restoration of microcirculatory flow is critical in calciphylaxis, where thrombosis contributes to dermal necrosis and subsequent tissue loss. Importantly, tPA demonstrates heightened efficacy in acidic microenvironments (pH < 7.0), a common characteristic of calciphylactic lesions due to local hypoxia.

A retrospective study evaluated the use of low-dose tissue plasminogen activator (tPA) as an adjunctive therapy for calciphylaxis by analyzing clinical outcomes in 15 patients treated at a tertiary care center. The findings indicated that while tPA did not result in a statistically significant increase in survival, it was associated with some improved outcomes and manageable safety concerns, including bleeding risks, within a multidisciplinary management approach that emphasized wound care and correction of calcium-phosphate balance [31]. However, a limited number of other retrospective studies did not show improvement on both lesion and survival [21, 32].

4.2.2 Direct oral anticoagulants (DOACs)

Direct oral anticoagulants (DOACs) selectively inhibit central enzymes in the coagulation cascade; apixaban and rivaroxaban target Factor Xa, while dabigatran inhibits thrombin. Their predictable pharmacokinetics and minimal drug-drug interactions have made them agents of choice in calciphylaxis, particularly among patients with end-stage renal disease (ESRD) on dialysis.

King et al. investigate the use of DOACs as an alternative to warfarin in patients with calciphylaxis. In this retrospective review of 16 patients with calciphylaxis treated with DOACs, the medications were found to be safe and well tolerated, with some patients experiencing improvement or complete resolution of their condition [33]. DOACs are contraindicated in patients with severe hepatic impairment (Child-Pugh Class C) or those receiving strong CYP3A4 inhibitors (e.g., ketoconazole). Renal dosing adjustments are necessary; for example, apixaban should be reduced to 2.5 mg twice daily in patients with serum creatinine ≥1.5 mg/dL [34]. The choice of DOAC should be guided by the degree of renal impairment and calls for randomized trials to further evaluate treatment efficacy.

4.2.3 Vitamin K supplementation

Vitamin K1 (phylloquinone) and vitamin K2 (menaquinones) are essential cofactors for γ-glutamyl carboxylase, enabling the carboxylation and activation of matrix Gla protein (MGP). The active, carboxylated form of MGP binds calcium ions and inhibits bone morphogenetic protein-2 (BMP-2)-mediated osteogenic differentiation of vascular smooth muscle cells. Case reports [35, 36] have documented significant improvement or resolution of calciphylaxis with high-dose vitamin K therapy (10 mg phylloquinone administered orally or intravenously three times per week). However, randomized controlled trials are needed to further assess the efficacy of this treatment approach.

4.3 Wound management: Bridging ischemia and infection

4.3.1 Hyperbaric oxygen therapy (HBOT)

HBOT at 2.4 atmospheres absolute (ATA) increases dissolved oxygen plasma concentration from 0.3 mL/dL to 6.8 mL/dL, enabling diffusion into hypoxic tissues beyond capillary dropout zones. This hyperoxia stimulates HIF-1α degradation, reducing VEGF-driven edema while enhancing neutrophil oxidative killing of *Pseudomonas aeruginosa*—a common pathogen in calciphylactic ulcers.

A few studies—including case series, retrospective reviews, and case reports—suggest that adjunctive HBOT may contribute to pain reduction, improved wound healing, and even increased survival rates in some calciphylaxis patients, though variability in efficacy and patient response is evident [37–39]. These findings highlight the need for more rigorous, large-scale studies to clarify HBOT's therapeutic role, optimal treatment protocols, and long-term outcomes in calciphylaxis management.

4.3.2 Amniotic mesenchymal stem cells (AMSCs)

AMSCs secrete exosomes containing miR-126-3p and miR-29a, which downregulate procalcific genes (e.g., RUNX2) in VSMCs while upregulating angiogenic factors (e.g., SDF-1α). This dual action reduces calcific debris and promotes neovascularization. Some reported the beneficial effect of MSC therapy in attenuating skin ulcerations and accelerating wound healing, which could serve as an intervention to ameliorate skin inflammatory conditions in the patients [40, 41].

4.3.3 Surgical debridement

Current knowledge highlights surgical debridement as an important component of multidisciplinary treatment strategies, often combined with interventions such as intensified hemodialysis, sodium thiosulfate infusion, and advanced wound care. Evidence from case reports and retrospective studies suggests that surgical debridement can aid wound healing and pain control, but optimal protocols remain unresolved due to the rarity and complexity of calciphylaxis [32, 42].

4.4 Pain management

Pain associated with calciphylaxis is often severe, persistent, and refractory to standard analgesic regimens, posing a major therapeutic challenge. Opioids are the cornerstone of pain control in calciphylaxis, as the majority of patients experience nociceptive and neuropathic pain that is severe and often requires escalation beyond nonopioid agents. Morphine, hydromorphone, and fentanyl are commonly utilized; fentanyl is often preferred in patients with advanced kidney dysfunction due to its pharmacokinetic profile and reduced accumulation of neurotoxic metabolites [43]. Methadone may be effective, particularly for mixed nociceptive-neuropathic pain, and offers the advantage of providing pain control in opioid-tolerant patients, but it requires expertise in dosing due to its variable half-life and risk of arrhythmias [44].

Adjuvant analgesics are frequently employed to address the neuropathic component of calciphylaxis pain. Gabapentin and pregabalin are anticonvulsants with proven efficacy for neuropathic pain, although dosing adjustments are critical due to their renal elimination [45]. Tricyclic antidepressants (e.g., amitriptyline) and serotonin-norepinephrine reuptake inhibitors (e.g., duloxetine) have theoretical benefit; however, evidence in calciphylaxis-specific populations is limited, and side effects must be carefully weighed.

In addition, acetaminophen can be a safe adjunct for mild-to-moderate pain and for its opioid-sparing effects, while nonsteroidal anti-inflammatory drugs (NSAIDs) are generally avoided due to renal toxicity [46]. Topical agents, such as lidocaine patches or eutectic mixtures (lidocaine-prilocaine), can provide localized relief, especially during dressing changes or minor procedures.

DOI: http://dx.doi.org/10.5772/intechopen.1011075

Given the frequency of refractory pain, consultation with palliative care or pain specialists is strongly recommended. Recent evidence also supports the use of novel interventions, such as peripheral nerve blocks and image-guided cryoneurolysis, particularly in intractable cases [47]. Given the complexity of pain in calciphylaxis, successful management is individualized, aiming not only for analgesia but also for optimal quality of life.

4.5 Multidisciplinary protocols: Synergizing expertise

A multidisciplinary protocol [40] for calciphylaxis management involves rapid diagnosis and collaborative interventions from nephrology, dermatology, wound care, palliative care, pain management, and nutrition teams. Nephrologists optimize dialysis—preferably daily or more frequent sessions—while strictly controlling calcium and phosphate balance, discontinuing triggering medications (e.g., warfarin, calcium-based binders, vitamin D analogs), and starting sodium thiosulfate as adjunctive therapy. Pain control is managed through a multimodal approach, prioritizing opioids and adjuvant analgesics, and considering regional anesthesia for refractory cases. Dermatology and wound teams promote non-adherent dressings, infection surveillance, selective surgical debridement, and negative pressure wound therapy as indicated. Dietary consultation supports protein and energy intake crucial for healing. Palliative care ensures expert symptom relief, supports complex decision-making, and addresses psychosocial needs early in care. Regular interdisciplinary meetings and personalized care plans are essential to adapt strategies over time and maximize patient outcomes.

The management of CUA remains one of the most challenging aspects of treating patients with end-stage renal disease. As current research highlights, the multifactorial nature of CUA demands an integrated approach that encompasses not only aggressive symptomatic management but also a deep dive into the molecular underpinnings of the disease. The development and validation of novel diagnostic biomarkers, combined with well-designed clinical trials, may eventually open the door to more effective, targeted therapies. Until then, multidisciplinary collaboration and personalized medicine will play pivotal roles in optimizing patient outcomes and advancing our understanding of this complex disorder.

By addressing these unresolved issues and by supporting collaborative, translational research efforts, the nephrology community can hope to move closer to a unified model of CUA pathogenesis. In turn, such advances will pave the way for the development of diagnostic tools and treatment protocols that can dramatically reduce the morbidity and mortality associated with this devastating condition.

Author details

Wen Wen
Department of Nephrology, Beijing Tsinghua Changgung Hospital, School of Clinical Medicine, Tsinghua Medicine, Tsinghua University, Beijing, China

*Address all correspondence to: wwa01275@btch.edu.cn

IntechOpen

© 2025 The Author(s). Licensee IntechOpen. This chapter is distributed under the terms of the Creative Commons Attribution License (http://creativecommons.org/licenses/by/4.0), which permits unrestricted use, distribution, and reproduction in any medium, provided the original work is properly cited.

References

[1] Angelis M et al. Calciphylaxis in patients on hemodialysis: A prevalence study. Surgery. 1997;**122**(6):1083-1089; discussion 1089-90

[2] Liu Y et al. Prevalence and clinical characteristics of Calciphylaxis in Chinese hemodialysis patients. Frontiers in Medicine (Lausanne). 2022;**9**:902171

[3] Ogah CO et al. Risk factors associated with the development of calciphylaxis in patients with chronic kidney disease: A systematic review. Cureus. 2024;**16**(12):e75314

[4] Dominguez AR. New debates surrounding the histopathological findings of calciphylaxis-do these give us new insights into pathogenesis of the disease? JAMA Dermatology. 2019;**155**(7):773-775

[5] Seethapathy H, Noureddine L. Calciphylaxis: Approach to diagnosis and management. Advances in Chronic Kidney Disease. 2019;**26**(6):484-490

[6] Wiltfang L, Booken N, Schneider SW. Successful novel treatment of nonuremic calciphylaxis with sodium thiosulfate and Iloprost: A case report. Case Reports in Dermatology. 2022;**14**(3):269-274

[7] Akad N et al. Calciphylaxis following parathyroidectomy in chronic kidney disease patients-case report and literature review. Biomedicine. 2025;**13**(3):1-13

[8] Ruderman I et al. Vascular calcification in skin and subcutaneous tissue in patients with chronic and end-stage kidney disease. BMC Nephrology. 2020;**21**(1):279

[9] Sowers KM, Hayden MR. Calcific uremic arteriolopathy: Pathophysiology, reactive oxygen species and therapeutic approaches. Oxidative Medicine and Cellular Longevity. 2010;**3**(2):109-121

[10] Wickens O et al. The role of iron in calciphylaxis-a current review. Journal of Clinical Medicine. 2022;**11**(19):1-8

[11] Jobbagy S et al. Multicenter evaluation of certainty and reliability in calciphylaxis diagnosis using a digital imaging platform. Laboratory Investigation. 2025;**105**(7):104169

[12] Dobry AS et al. Association between hypercoagulable conditions and calciphylaxis in patients with renal disease: A case-control study. JAMA Dermatology. 2018;**154**(2):182-187

[13] Napoleon MA et al. Activation and targetability of TYMP-IL-6-TF signaling in the skin microenvironment in uremic calciphylaxis. Science Translational Medicine. 2025;**17**(795):eadn5772

[14] Wolner Z et al. Redefining calciphylaxis as a uniquely bone forming subcutaneous C5b-9-mediated microvascular injury syndrome associated with localized subcutaneous and systemic complement pathway activation. The American Journal of Dermatopathology. 2024;**46**(12):807-818

[15] Ketteler M, Brandenburg VM. K-alcification protection in dialysis patients: The underestimated phenomenon of vitamin K deficiency. Journal of the American Society of Nephrology. 2017;**28**(6):1667-1668

[16] Hasegawa H. Clinical assessment of warfarin therapy in patients with maintenance dialysis-clinical efficacy, risks and development of calciphylaxis.

Annals of Vascular Diseases. 2017;**10**(3):170-177

[17] Rothe H et al. Ecto-5′ -Nucleotidase CD73 (NT5E), vitamin D receptor and FGF23 gene polymorphisms may play a role in the development of calcific uremic arteriolopathy in dialysis patients - data from the German Calciphylaxis registry. PLoS One. 2017;**12**(2):e0172407

[18] Musso CG et al. Differential diagnosis of calciphylaxis in chronic dialysis patients. International Urology and Nephrology. 2020;**52**(3):595-597

[19] Dusing P et al. Vascular pathologies in chronic kidney disease: Pathophysiological mechanisms and novel therapeutic approaches. Journal of Molecular Medicine (Berlin, Germany). 22 January 2021

[20] Groover M, Nutan F. Role of bone scan in diagnosis of calciphylaxis: A review. JAAD International. 2024;**14**:31-33

[21] McCarthy JT et al. Survival, risk factors, and effect of treatment in 101 patients with calciphylaxis. Mayo Clinic Proceedings. 2016;**91**(10):1384-1394

[22] Liu Y, Zhang X. Early diagnosis strategy of calciphylaxis in dialysis patients. Renal Failure. 2023;**45**(2):2264407

[23] Peng T et al. Systematic review of sodium thiosulfate in treating calciphylaxis in chronic kidney disease patients. Nephrology (Carlton). 2018;**23**(7):669-675

[24] Nigwekar SU et al. Sodium thiosulfate therapy for calcific uremic arteriolopathy. Clinical Journal of the American Society of Nephrology. 2013;**8**(7):1162-1170

[25] Yang X et al. Use of the optimized sodium thiosulfate regimen for the treatment of calciphylaxis in Chinese patients. Renal Failure. 2022;**44**(1):914-922

[26] Strazzula L et al. Intralesional sodium thiosulfate for the treatment of calciphylaxis. JAMA Dermatology. 2013;**149**(8):946-949

[27] Wen W et al. Intravenous sodium thiosulphate for calciphylaxis of chronic kidney disease: A systematic review and meta-analysis. JAMA Network Open. 2023;**6**(4):e2310068

[28] Sinha S et al. The CALCIPHYX study: A randomized, double-blind, placebo-controlled, phase 3 clinical trial of SNF472 for the treatment of calciphylaxis. Clinical Kidney Journal. 2022;**15**(1):136-144

[29] Sinha S et al. Hexasodium fytate for the treatment of calciphylaxis: A randomised, double-blind, phase 3, placebo-controlled trial with an open-label extension. E Clinical Medicine. 2024;**75**:102784

[30] Sewell LD et al. Low-dose tissue plasminogen activator for calciphylaxis. Archives of Dermatology. 2004;**140**(9):1045-1048

[31] El-Azhary RA et al. Retrospective analysis of tissue plasminogen activator as an adjuvant treatment for calciphylaxis. JAMA Dermatology. 2013;**149**(1):63-67

[32] Wen W et al. Patient-reported and clinical outcomes among patients with calciphylaxis. Mayo Clinic Proceedings: Innovations, Quality and Outcomes. 2023;**7**(1):81-92

[33] King BJ et al. Direct oral anticoagulant medications in

calciphylaxis. International Journal of Dermatology. 2017;**56**(10):1065-1070

[34] Fudim M et al. Apixaban dose in patients with atrial fibrillation and acute coronary syndrome and/or undergoing percutaneous coronary intervention: Insights from AUGUSTUS. JACC: Advances. 2025;**4**(4):101665

[35] Wajih Z, Singer R. Successful treatment of calciphylaxis with vitamin K in a patient on haemodialysis. Clinical Kidney Journal. 2022;**15**(2):354-356

[36] Christiadi D, Singer RF. Calciphylaxis in a dialysis patient successfully treated with high-dose vitamin K supplementation. Clinical Kidney Journal. 2018;**11**(4):528-529

[37] Brekke FB et al. Hyperbaric oxygen treatment in addition to conventional multidisciplinary care in patients with calciphylaxis. Clinical Nephrology. 2025;**103**(1):1-4

[38] Pathault E et al. Hyperbaric oxygen therapy enables pain reduction and healing in painful chronic wounds, including in calciphylaxis. Annales de Dermatologie et de Vénéréologie. 2024;**151**(4):103325

[39] Biglione B et al. A retrospective review of outcomes after hyperbaric oxygen therapy for the treatment of calciphylaxis. Journal of the American Academy of Dermatology. 2024;**90**(1):45-51

[40] Pan Y et al. The application of MDT model for calciphylaxis management in patients with end-stage renal disease. International Wound Journal. 2023;**20**(9):3717-3723

[41] Bhamidipati T et al. Beneficial effects of amnion-chorion stem cell grafting in the long term management of nonuremic calciphylaxis wounds. Cureus. 2020;**12**(12):e12170

[42] Wipattanakitcharoen A, Takkavatakarn K, Susantitaphong P. Risk factors, treatment modalities, and clinical outcomes of penile calciphylaxis: Systematic review. World Journal of Urology. 2023;**41**(11):2959-2966

[43] Kurniawan HI et al. Calciphylaxis and intractable pain in a veteran with psychological trauma history. Journal of Palliative Medicine. 2024;**27**(9):1279-1283

[44] King SJ, Kondasinghe JS. Treatment of painful calciphylaxis with methadone in a palliative care unit: A case report. Clinical Nephrology – Case Studies. 2023;**11**:6-11

[45] Karmegam S, Shetty A. Calciphylaxis after parathyroidectomy. Hemodialysis International. 2017;**21**(Suppl. 2):S62-S66

[46] Kodumudi V et al. Management of cutaneous calciphylaxis. Advances in Therapy. 2020;**37**(12):4797-4807

[47] Edquist MK, Azene EM. Image-guided peripheral nerve cryoneurolysis for pain relief in calciphylaxis. Journal of Vascular and Interventional Radiology. 2020;**31**(11):1947-1949

Chapter 6

Long-Term Hemodialysis Access: How to Determine and Perform It?

Yunanto Kurnia, Trianingsih and Maura Andini Setiabudi

Abstract

Chronic kidney disease (CKD) is an escalating global health issue, affecting more than 10% of the global population, with obesity and diabetes as significant risk factors. As CKD advances to end-stage kidney disease (ESKD), patients frequently require kidney replacement therapy (KRT), primarily hemodialysis. The selection of vascular access, including central venous catheter (CVC), arteriovenous fistula (AVF), or graft (AVG), is essential for long-term dialysis success. This chapter explores the fundamentals of hemodialysis (HD) access selection, preoperative evaluation, and management, emphasizing the value of personalized assessment. Furthermore, this chapter elaborates on several access strategies with the objective of optimizing long-term access function and reducing complications throughout the patient's dialysis experience.

Keywords: chronic kidney disease, hemodialysis access, vascular access planning, arteriovenous fistula, arteriovenous graft, basilic vein transposition

1. Introduction

Chronic kidney disease (CKD) is a significant growing global health challenge, affecting more than 10% of the population worldwide. Its prevalence continues to rise owing to common risk factors, such as obesity and diabetes mellitus (DM). As CKD progresses to end-stage kidney disease (ESKD), patients may require lifelong kidney replacement therapy (KRT), which represents a substantial burden, especially in low- and middle-income countries [1]. The Kidney Disease Outcomes Quality Initiative (KDOQI) 2019 guidelines recommend the estimation of glomerular filtration rate (GFR) as a critical tool for both diagnosis and management. Ideally, a CKD patient with an estimated GFR of 15–20 mL/min/1.73 m^2 will have been properly educated about KRT modalities and future treatment planning to facilitate informed decision-making [2]. Among the available KRT modalities, long-term hemodialysis remains essential for this population. The management of this therapy requires careful consideration, including vascular access choice, site selection, and patient-specific factors, ensuring lifetime, continual functioning dialysis access that minimizes complications. The optimal choice of vascular access includes central venous catheter (CVC), arteriovenous fistula (AVF), or graft (AVG) [3]. In urgent or emergent dialysis initiation, patients often begin treatment *via* CVC due to its convenient placement.

However, once stabilized, long-term and more durable vascular access must be carefully considered. This chapter will discuss the principles of selecting, planning, and managing long-term hemodialysis access to optimize patient outcomes over the course of therapy.

2. Preoperative evaluation

Preoperative evaluation involves a comprehensive assessment of patient-specific factors and vascular anatomy. This process is a crucial step in planning hemodialysis vascular access, aiming to create long-term access. It ensures that the chosen access method will provide optimal function and durability.

2.1 Risk factors

A thorough evaluation of the patient's medical history is crucial in predicting future AV access patency. Several factors, including age, sex, and comorbidities, contribute to the pathophysiology of the arterial and venous systems, thus affecting access longevity. In a study by Yoshida et al. [4] involving 611 patients, aging, female sex, and diabetes mellitus (DM) are identified as significant risk factors for AV access dysfunction, as reflected in 24-month primary patency rates. The median age of participants involved was 70 years, and nearly half were undergoing dialysis due to diabetes. Aging and DM are associated with poorer overall health conditions, while females are reported to have a smaller vascular diameter compared to males, thereby potentially increasing access complications. Similar findings by Garcia-Lopez et al. [5] and Long et al. [6] identified age over 60 years, female sex, and diabetes as key predictors of AV access failure. An earlier study by De Pinho et al. [7] also confirmed that age, gender, DM, and primary renal disease, including hypertension and diabetic nephropathy, are significantly correlated with decreased AV access patency. Taken together, all of these factors must be thoroughly evaluated to guide the selection of AV access and anticipate any potential complications following surgery.

2.2 Vascular anatomy assessment

Among many factors, the patient's vascular anatomy is the key predictor influencing the ideal type and location of access. This process includes a comprehensive clinical examination and vascular imaging *via* duplex ultrasound (DUS). A detailed physical examination of the arterial system, venous system, and general cardiovascular evaluation serves as the initial step in predicting the vascular characteristics of the patient [2]. In certain populations, such as obese patients, where physical examination alone may be challenging, vascular imaging plays a crucial role in vascular access creation. Vascular imaging plays a pivotal role in the preoperative evaluation for vascular access creation. The purpose of this assessment is to identify suitable veins and arteries that are capable of supporting a long-term, durable access site and also ensuring procedural success.

Duplex ultrasound remains the preferred noninvasive modality for preoperative vessel mapping due to its accessibility, safety, and cost-effectiveness. It offers real-time assessment of the vessel diameter, depth, and flow as parameters for AVF maturation, which will be further discussed later. DUS also helps identify potential stenosis or obstruction that could compromise access patency. In line with this, the

KDOQI 2019 guidelines recommend routine preoperative vessel mapping using DUS in patients at high risk of AV access failure to improve AVF outcomes. In addition, more advanced imaging techniques may be required in cases when ultrasound is inconclusive or when further detailed imaging is needed [8]. Computed tomography angiography (CTA) provides high spatial resolution of the surrounding vessel structure and is often reserved for complex anatomy cases. However, it carries risks related to radiation exposure and iodinated contrast agent exposure, which can be nephrotoxic and contraindicated in some patients. Digital subtraction angiography (DSA) and venography (DSV) are considered the gold standard for visualization of the arterial and venous vasculature, which allows identification of an occult central venous stenotic disease and occlusion. Although invasive, DSA allows for immediate intervention. Similar to CTA, this modality also possesses the risk of radiation and contrast exposure. Lastly, magnetic resonance angiography (MRA) provides high-resolution images, particularly for small and medium-sized vessels that may be difficult to visualize with CTA or DSA. MRA can be chosen when radiation exposure is a concern.

3. Overview of hemodialysis access

Patients with CKD who are either preparing to initiate hemodialysis, transitioning from another kidney replacement modality, or already on hemodialysis with a failing access will need consideration for hemodialysis vascular access. However, the actual need for hemodialysis access modalities depends on the patient's current individualized ESKD care plan. This care plan should encompass continuous care for a specific patient's current medical situation, future therapy goals, chosen modality for kidney replacement therapy (KRT), preferences, social support, functional status, and other practical feasibilities. As a case example, a patient undergoing regular hemodialysis *via* right internal jugular (RIJ) vein catheter (*in situ* for 13 days) with a history of diabetes mellitus presented with recurrent chills during dialysis and leukocytosis, which strongly suggests a catheter-related bloodstream infection (CRBSI). As infection may arise *via* the catheter lumen despite a clean exit site, prompt catheter removal and reinsertion at a new site are recommended, alongside empirical antibiotic therapy. Due to the necessity for continuous dialysis, long-term vascular access must be taken into account. Ultrasound mapping revealed suitable vessels in the distal left arm for arteriovenous fistula (AVF) creation, with cephalic vein and radial artery diameters >2 mm and no signs of atherosclerosis. However, as AVF maturation requires at least six weeks, a temporary catheter should be placed in the right femoral vein to minimize the risk of infection and central venous stenosis. In this scenario, the insertion of a new catheter into the right internal jugular or subclavian vein presents a considerable risk of recurrent infection and central venous stenosis. Furthermore, positioning both the AVF and temporary catheter on the same side heightens the risk of ipsilateral upper limb edema. Consequently, the suitable management strategy is commencing AVF formation in the distal left arm while transferring the HD catheter to the right femoral vein as a provisional access site. Moreover, it is essential to initiate hand-strengthening exercises—such as consistently lifting a 1 kg weight—to enhance vascular growth. In this scenario, a well-developed right arm would serve as an appropriate location for future arteriovenous fistula creation, guaranteeing continued access for long-term dialysis if renal transplantation is not practical (**Figures 1–3**).

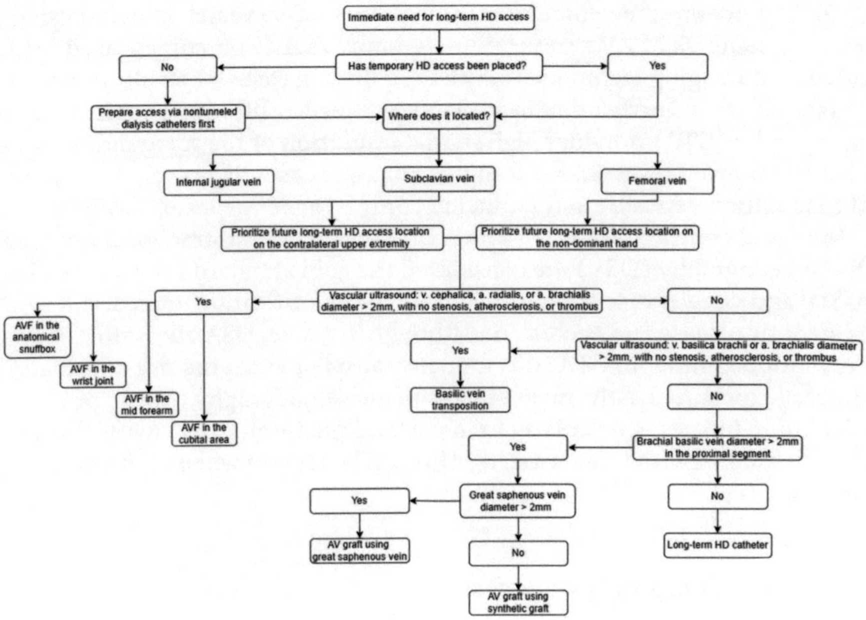

Figure 1.
Yunanto rule 1: Algorithm for immediate long-term hemodialysis (HD) access planning based on patient condition and potential vascular access sites.

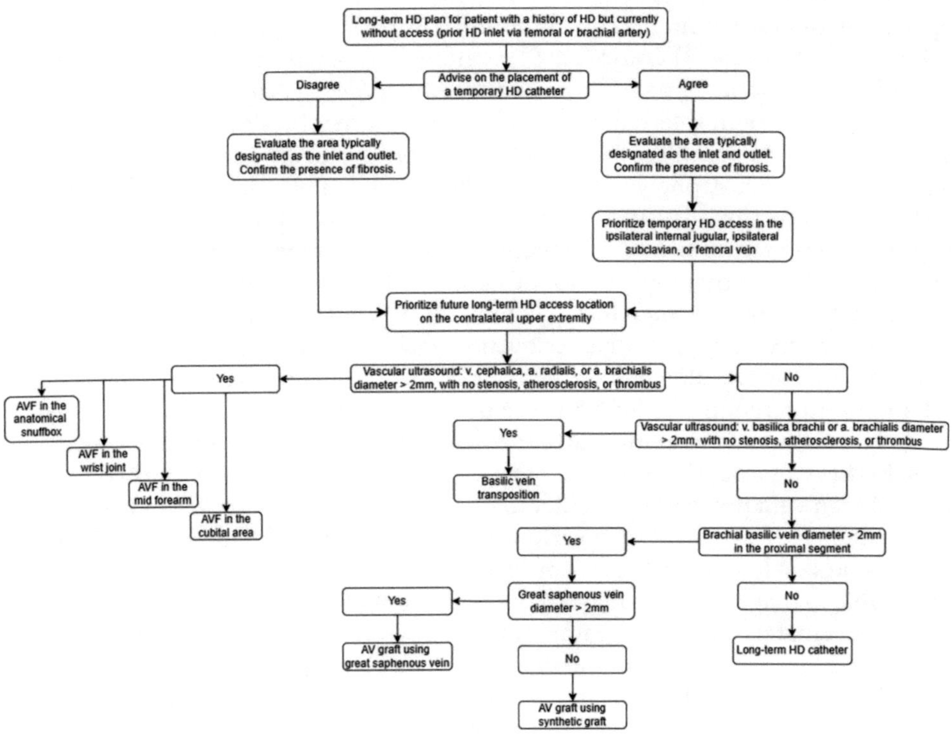

Figure 2.
Yunanto rule 2: Algorithm for long-term HD access planning in patients with a history of HD.

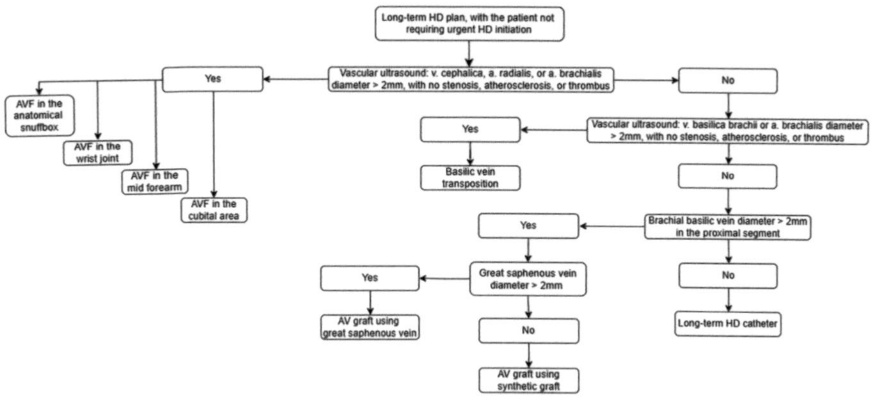

Figure 3.
Yunanto rule 3: Algorithm for long-term HD access planning for patients not requiring urgent HD initiation.

3.1 Central venous catheter

More than 80% of patients initiate their hemodialysis program with a central venous catheter. CVCs for hemodialysis can be classified based on their intended duration of use: acute and chronic. Acute or nontunneled dialysis catheters (NTDCs) are associated with a higher risk of infectious complications and are prone to dislodgement; thus, they should only be placed in hospitalized patients and used for a short duration, usually less than 2 weeks. According to KDOQI 2019, NTDC is acceptable for short-term dialysis, including patients with AVF or AVG created but not ready to use, dysfunction of previous vascular access, and in need of short-term use of dialysis [9]. In contrast, chronic or tunneled dialysis catheters (TDCs) are suitable for outpatient use and can remain for extended periods. Long-term use of TDCs is typically indicated in patients with multiple prior failed AV accesses, limited life expectancy, absence of AV access creation options due to inflow artery or outflow vein problems, or patient preference.

3.1.1 Preprocedural consideration

Prior to placement, a comprehensive preoperative evaluation is essential. This begins with a detailed review of the patient's medical history, including prior long-term central line placement, prior AVF or AVG placement, prior TDC-related infections, coagulation disorder, and pacemaker implantation. Repeated use of central lines may lead to scarring, stenosis, and thrombosis, which can complicate future catheter insertions. Additionally, a physical examination of the neck and chest should be done to evaluate local anatomical changes, upper extremity or facial edema, and ipsilateral venous distention with venous collaterals to alert to the possibility of central venous occlusive disease. For central venous imaging, noninvasive color-flow DUS is the first-line imaging modality. As mentioned above, it facilitates prompt evaluation of the patency, venous pressure, and thrombus presence.

3.1.2 Site selection

Upper extremity access is preferred over lower extremity access whenever it is clinically feasible. For long-term access, the recommended order of preferred insertion sites is internal jugular, femoral, and lastly, subclavian veins. The right internal jugular (RIJ) vein is typically favored over the left internal jugular (LIJ) vein due to its superior patency, presumably owing to its shorter and more direct course to the superior vena cava and less risk of kinking [10]. However, possible anatomical anomalies like persistent left superior vena cava anomalies should be considered to avoid complications. As noted in the algorithm (**Figure 1**), placing the upper extremity catheter on the contralateral side to the planned permanent AV access is recommended to preserve the central veins on the access side. Ipsilateral catheter placement is associated with an increased risk of venous stenosis and thrombosis, which may impair outflow from the AVF or AVG, leading to access failure. This was caused by endothelial injury due to microthrombi formation, smooth muscle proliferation, and venous wall remodeling that may progress to venous stenosis and occlusion. In the end, this may negatively affect AV access maturation and patency. Studies show that contralateral catheter placement is associated with better vascular access outcomes and longer access survival [11, 12]. Therefore, placing the CVC contralateral to the planned AV access preserves the venous outflow tract on the future access side. If not feasible, the femoral vein may be considered as an alternative, although several important factors must be evaluated. Femoral access should be avoided in patients with a higher body mass index (BMI), as a previous study has demonstrated a significant risk of catheter colonization with a BMI greater than 28.4 [13]. This heightened risk is likely attributed to challenges in maintaining catheter site hygiene and increased skin fold depth, which increases the risk of bacterial overgrowth. In selected circumstances, femoral CVC preserves central veins to ensure the feasibility of future AV access placement. Lastly, subclavian vein access should be avoided if possible due to its high association with catheter-induced subclavian stenosis, which may affect future placement of ipsilateral permanent AV access [9].

CVC insertion is associated with various complications, broadly categorized into mechanical, infectious, and thrombotic events. Previous meta-analysis by Marik et al. [14] showed that there is no significant difference in infectious and thrombotic complications between jugular, femoral, and subclavian vein access. However, a more recent study by Sakuraya et al. [15] showed a lesser risk of infectious complications for subclavian access compared with jugular access. These evolving insights into the risks associated with different insertion sites highlight the need for individualized patient care in the selection of optimal catheter sites.

3.2 Arteriovenous fistula

An arteriovenous fistula is considered the most durable form of VA for hemodialysis, associated with the longest patency and lowest rates of complications compared with AVG and CVC. An autologous AVF is created through a surgical anastomosis between an artery and a vein, which diverts the high-flow arterial blood into the low-pressure vein, resulting in remodeling of the vein, which lowers shear stress by increasing luminal diameter and hoop stress by increasing wall thickness of the vein [16]. This process, known as arterialization, will eventually result in the maturation of the fistula, allowing it to support hemodialysis. AVF requires approximately 6 weeks to mature, although approximately 25–30% of AVFs never achieve maturation [17–19]. Multiple factors contributed to the maturation process, such as diabetes, hypertension, peripheral vascular disease, smoking, endothelial dysfunction, and vein diameter [18, 20]. Given this variable, AVFs ideally should be created 3–6 months prior to the anticipated time of use to allow sufficient time for maturation and any potential surgical revision.

3.2.1 Preprocedural consideration

It is important to acknowledge that the AVF failure rate is still alarmingly high, with maturation presenting a significant challenge in over 50% of cases. Therefore, preoperative arterial and venous mapping is crucial to maximize the chances of successful and durable access. Previous studies show that perioperative mapping results in higher immediate success rates, improves access adequacy, and prevents unnecessary delays in future treatment plans [19, 21]. As mentioned above, vein diameter constitutes one of the most important factors for AV access maturation. To assess vein diameter, a phlebotomy tourniquet is applied for 1–2 minutes to the forearm and arm, depending on the vein location. This helps enlarge the vein, thus resulting in a greater number of patients qualifying for AVF creation. Following this, a detailed assessment is carried out using DUS, documenting the inner diameter and the depth of the vein along its path [22]. While different centers may apply varying vein diameter thresholds, a minimum vein diameter of 2 mm is generally preferred for optimal access, as veins below this size are more likely to experience poor maturation and higher failure rates. Meta-analyses by Feng et al. [23], Aljarrah et al. [19], and Kordzadeh et al. [24] support this by showing that veins larger than 2 mm exhibit a significantly higher functional maturation rate. Similarly, arterial diameter is routinely assessed at the level of the intended anastomosis. It is essential to evaluate not only the diameter but also the presence of atherosclerotic plaques and calcification, as these can increase the risk of future complications, including thrombosis or pseudoaneurysm formation. Pseudoaneurysms can occur when repeated puncture leads to the disruption of the vessel wall. For the artery, a diameter over 2 mm also correlates with superior maturation and better long-term patency [24, 25]. Therefore, ensuring both venous and arterial diameters meet minimum thresholds is critical to ensure a functional and lasting AVF that is capable of withstanding the high blood flow demands of hemodialysis.

3.2.2 Site selection

As mentioned before, due to easier accessibility and lower infection rates, upper extremity access is preferred over lower extremity, with the nondominant arm as the first choice, unless the mapping indicates unsuitable vessels in that extremity. The nondominant hand is often chosen for access insertion to minimize the risk of complications associated with physical activity [23]. The dominant hand is being used more frequently for various tasks that may result in increased mechanical stress on the vascular access and increase the risk of access site trauma. Placing the access in the nondominant hand allows for better movement, enabling the patient to continue with their previous daily activities without risking interfering with the function of the dialysis access. However, previous studies and guidelines have underscored the importance of upper limb exercise in promoting vascular remodeling, a process essential for optimizing AVF maturation and long-term usability [2, 26]. Postoperative hand isometric exercises have been shown to promote both clinical maturation and functional patency of the AVF by promoting increased blood flow, vein dilation, and wall thickening, thus improving the vessel's suitability for repeated cannulation [26]. If possible, AV access should be placed as distally as possible to preserve the veins of the proximal sites for future access if needed [2, 27]. Distal sites also have a lower risk of steal syndrome, as the diversion of blood flow is less likely to affect the distal tissues significantly, owing to smaller vein size and the presence of collateral circulation. This risk is relatively higher in patients with diabetes and the elderly, who may already have compromised vascular health [28]. Therefore, the cephalic vein is often the preferred choice for AVF creation due to its superficial and lateral location, which allows for easier access. As mentioned above and in the algorithm, at least 2 mm of vein diameter is required for choosing this access. The anatomical snuffbox is often the first choice as it has the best proximity to the posterior branch of the radial artery and cephalic vein, which are ideal for creating access with minimal risk of complications. If the posterior branch of the radial artery is considered inadequate but the radial artery is still adequate, wrist access is chosen to create a radiocephalic fistula. If the wrist area is considered unsuitable, the mid-forearm, approximately four fingers or 8–10 cm above the wrist, can be selected as an alternative site. At this location, two superficial veins are typically encountered: the accessory cephalic vein and the cephalic vein. The accessory cephalic vein can present significant challenges when creating radiocephalic AVF access. The presence of this vein, particularly those that divert blood from the primary cephalic vein, is linked to poor maturation of the fistula. Studies by Lin et al. [29] indicate that when the accessory vein diameter exceeds 80% of the cephalic vein diameter, it will become a competing outflow pathway and further hinder proper maturation. Studies have demonstrated that ligation significantly improves maturation rates. Radiocephalic fistulas have higher rates of long-term patency than those at other sites. However, when the distal cephalic vein is considered insufficient due to factors such as inadequate size or other anatomical limitations, the accessory cephalic vein may be used instead. This technique is particularly useful when the accessory cephalic vein and the proximal cephalic vein are sufficiently large and meet the minimum diameter threshold. Instead of solely relying on the distal cephalic vein, ligating it and redirecting blood flow to the accessory cephalic vein can be a viable option. While this approach is not widely documented, it may be considered based on clinical experience and individual patient anatomy (**Figure 4**).

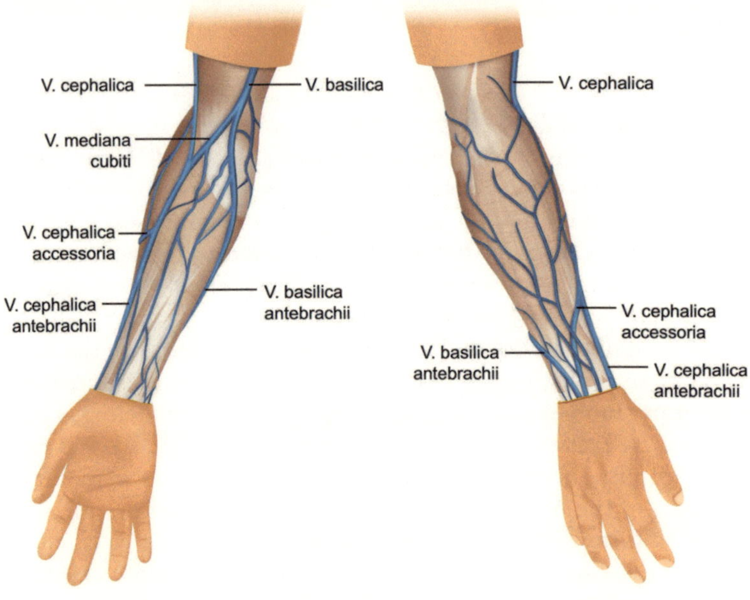

Figure 4.
Illustration of forearm vein anatomy. The cephalic vein is the most common vein used for hemodialysis access due to its location on the lateral side. Alternatively, the accessory cephalic vein, located in the mid-forearm area, may also be utilized.

In patients unsuitable for radiocephalic fistula creation, a more proximal fistula, such as the brachiocephalic AVF at the antecubital fossa, is the next option [2, 27] Compared to the radiocephalic, the brachiocephalic fistula has faster maturation times due to greater blood flow but is more difficult to create, has higher rates of distal ischemia, and is associated with stenosis of the cephalic arch [16]. Lastly, if the cephalic vein is not adequate, transposition of the basilic vein is considered as an alternative. Compared to AVG, basilic vein transposition offers better primary and secondary patency. Moreover, the use of saphenous vein graft (SVG) conduit for AVG is generally deferred as a last option, as it ensures that the lower extremities remain available for future temporary hemodialysis catheter in the event of failing primary AVF access. This is also supported by the KDOQI 2019 guideline, which recommends the use of autogenous fistula over grafts whenever possible due to their superior patency, lower infection rates, and reduced need for interventions [2]. For the arterial access, the distal radial artery, ulnar artery, proximal radial artery, and brachial artery can be chosen, starting from the distal part to preserve more proximal sites. The Allen test is an essential procedure to evaluate the patency of the radial and ulnar arteries, ensuring adequate collateral circulation before creating an AVF, which is particularly important to prevent steal syndrome. By performing this test, the clinician can confirm that the ulnar artery provides sufficient collateral flow if the radial artery is used for the fistula, thereby reducing the risk of ischemia.

3.2.3 Monitoring and complications

All AVFs should undergo clinical evaluation at 6–8 weeks after creation to assess for signs of maturation. Key clinical indicators include the presence of a strong thrill and a sufficiently dilated vein, ideally 8–10 cm in length and at least 6 mm in diameter, with a superficial course. If not possible, maturation can be determined using the "Rule of 6's" of sonographic criteria, including outflow vein diameter $\geq$ 6 mm, outflow vein depth $\leq$ 6 mm, and blood flow >600 mL/min [16]. This adequate size and superficiality are necessary for ensuring that the fistula is suitable for routine cannulation and can provide effective dialysis. Once an AVF has matured, several strategies for AVF maintenance are crucial to preserve access function and prevent complications. This includes regular assessment for a thrill, avoidance of blood pressure measurement on the AVF arm, and prohibition of venipuncture or catheter insertion into the outflow vein or other ipsilateral veins to preserve them for future access use. However, the risk of complications following AVF placement is still worth considering. As mentioned above, the most common complications include failure to mature, stenosis, thrombosis, infection, steal syndrome, and aneurysm formation [28, 30] According to the available guidelines, clopidogrel may be given for up to six months to improve fistula patency [2, 31]. Education for both healthcare providers and patients is essential to reinforce best practices for AVF care. Early detection and timely intervention are key to ensuring long-term patency and successful dialysis.

3.3 Arteriovenous graft

In cases where an arteriovenous fistula cannot be placed, either due to inadequate vein diameter, unfavorable anatomy, or previous access failures, a graft serves as an alternative hemodialysis access. An AVG is a vascular conduit that is surgically implanted to connect the arterial and venous circulation. Compared to the AVF, the AVG offers a quicker maturation time, approximately usable within 3–4 weeks, but is often associated with poor patient survival and higher complication rates, including infection, thrombosis, and graft failure, which negatively impact patient survival and quality of life [32, 33]. Despite these risks, AVGs provide a necessary alternative for patients requiring dialysis access with limited vascular access options.

3.3.1 Preprocedural consideration

For optimal AVG access creation, a clinical evaluation of the upper limb is necessary. The presence of superficial and collateral veins that imply a central vein occlusion, the presence of peripheral pulses, and skin integrity should be evaluated. Similar to AVF, DUS examination for arterial and venous mapping is necessary to reduce the need for secondary surgical or endovascular procedures. DUS provides a picture of arterial patency by the presence of stenosis or occlusions. An outflow study is needed to evaluate vessel patency and diameter, which are predictive factors of failure.

3.3.2 Graft access

Similar to AVFs, AVGs are ideally placed as distally in the arm as possible, where an adequate artery is identified. According to the current guidelines, common graft configurations for hemodialysis include the forearm loop, upper arm straight or curved, and upper arm looped [34]. For forearm access, the first option is radial-antecubital straight access, followed by brachial-antecubital looped access. When forearm vessels are deemed inadequate and upper arm access is required, proximal radial-axillary or brachial-axillary straight access may be considered. However, the impact and role of graft configuration on overall patency remain underexplored. A study by Mousa et al. [35] reported that neither graft location nor configuration significantly affects the primary patency of AVGs. Some suggest that this finding allows for greater flexibility in surgical decision-making, as the surgeon can decide the optimal graft configuration based on individual patient anatomy and clinical conditions without being constrained to the current guidelines.

AV access can be created using a variety of AVGs, including synthetic and autologous materials. Based on clinical settings and guidelines, SVG remains preferred over synthetic grafts, balancing its durability and infection risk. The ideal graft material should closely resemble the native vessels in terms of functionality and structure and also be nonthrombogenic, immunologically inert, resistant to infection and puncture trauma, and cost-effective. The greater saphenous vein can be used as an AVG conduit but has generally not given promising patency rates, which are 20% at 2 years. There is an increased operating time for saphenous vein harvesting, delayed healing of the thigh wound, and the need to preserve it for coronary arterial revascularization [36]. However, SVG is more cost-effective long-term due to the smaller risk of infection-related hospitalizations [37]. Over the years, expanded polytetrafluoroethylene (ePTFE) has become the gold standard graft material due to its good long-term patency, biocompatibility, and lower risk of complications. Other advantages of using PTFE grafts are short maturation time, typically 3–4 weeks, and multiple potential access sites. However, it is also associated with endothelial and fibromuscular hyperplasia, which can lead to venous outflow stenosis and subsequent thrombosis. A study by Halbert et al. [38] reported primary patency rates for ePTFE grafts of 56% at 6 months and 28% at 24 months. In the last few decades, various improvements have been made to improve their functionality, including covalent heparin bonding on the luminal surface and the use of self-sealing technologies. However, looking at the primary patency rates, despite the advanced growth of graft innovation, ePTFE grafts still exhibit relatively high failure rates, with nearly half of all ePTFE grafts failing within 2 years and requiring further treatment. A study by Yousef et al. [37] reported that, although statistically insignificant, ePTFE grafts demonstrated superior outcomes in terms of operative efficiency, maturation times, patency rates, and thrombosis incidence compared to saphenous vein grafts. However, PTFE use was associated with a higher risk of infection and pseudoaneurysm formation. Due to this benefit-to-risk ratio, the SVG conduit is preferable over the synthetic graft, and PTFE serves as a favorable alternative in cases where an autologous conduit is not optimal.

3.3.3 Monitoring and complications

Postprocedural antiplatelet therapy (APT) is recommended following AVG creation to improve graft patency, with aspirin and P2Y12 inhibitors, such as clopidogrel, showing significant benefits. Studies by Ebertz et al. [39] and Locham et al. [40] indicate that single antiplatelet therapy (SAPT) increases 1-year primary patency rates from 44 to 48% and reduces thrombosis risk by 20%. On the other hand, dual antiplatelet therapy (DAPT) may further enhance outcomes, with a 24% lower risk of primary patency loss compared to zero APT, though it was associated with higher bleeding risk, thus necessitating cautious use. Clinical monitoring of bleeding risks is essential during therapy. Patients on DAPT should be regularly assessed for signs of spontaneous bleeding, and therapy should be adjusted accordingly. Prophylactic strategies such as patient education on avoiding trauma, meticulous cannulation techniques, and regular surveillance can mitigate bleeding complications. Current guidelines suggest low-dose aspirin and dipyridamole as first-line and reserving DAPT for higher-thrombosis-risk patients, balancing the efficacy against bleeding complications [2].

Routine postoperative surveillance plays a pivotal role in optimizing AVG outcomes. A study by Yen et al. [41] documented the importance of routine clinical surveillance of AVG patency, especially in patients with previous access complications. The most common complications associated with the use of AVG are stenosis and thrombosis of the venous outflow and graft infection. As mentioned above, venous stenosis and thrombosis are linked to cellular hyperplasia resulting from the compliance mismatch between the vein and graft. This incidence was found to be higher in males than females, explained by male cases being associated with more comorbidities and smoking [42]. Routine surveillance using DUS plays a vital role in detecting early stenosis, thrombosis, or flow abnormalities before clinical symptoms arise, allowing timely interventions. Besides stenosis and thrombosis, infections also pose a severe threat to AVG patency. Compared to AVF, infection in AVG occurs 10 times more frequently and is often associated with dialysis access closure. The synthetic material of ePTFE, although durable, provides a substrate prone to bacterial colonization, making infections challenging to eradicate and often necessitating graft removal. The overall infection rate of ePTFE graft infections is 9% per patient-year, underscoring the need for cautious aseptic techniques during cannulation and aggressive treatment of early infectious signs [38].

Overall, the integration of tailored antiplatelet therapy, vigilant surveillance utilizing DUS, and prompt management of complications is essential to prolong graft function. The multifactorial nature of AVG failure requires a multidisciplinary approach to optimize outcomes and minimize the morbidity associated with dialysis access failure.

4. Techniques and procedures for access creation

A careful, methodical approach tailored to each patient's vascular anatomy and condition is essential to ensure the longevity and functionality of the vascular access, as suboptimal surgical technique may lead to various complications, such as thrombosis and inadequate blood flow. Here, we are going to cover the procedural technique and common pitfalls for AVF and AVG placement.

The process of AVF access creation generally includes skin incision, vein identification and access, artery identification and access, and anastomosis creation. Common pitfalls, such as improper vessel selection and poor anastomotic technique, may negatively impact the outcome. This discussion will delve into the recommended techniques for AV fistula creation and explore key surgical strategies to avoid these pitfalls. Although each AVF access creation is unique, several principles can be broadly applied. After ensuring the anatomy with ultrasound Doppler, the surgeon should mark the course of the vein that will be accessed. For forearm access, the skin incision should be made with a lateral-to-medial orientation, running diagonally along the radial side of the forearm, with the patient's hand placed in a supine position. This incision technique provides optimal vein exposure, as it allows for better visualization of a longer segment of the vein, thus minimizing the risk of arterial kinking or vessel injury. For snuffbox access, to better expose the cephalic vein, position the hand with the palm facing the body. This positioning allows the surgeon to locate the vein without the need to dissect extensively toward the dorsal side. However, this technique may not be suitable if the goal is to use the accessory cephalic vein, as it runs on the dorsal side. Once identified, circumferentially dissect the vein to separate it from adjacent structures, ensuring it is fully mobilized and free to move without tension. In addition to evaluating the primary vein, it is essential to examine the branches of the selected vessel. It is recommended to ligate the branch vessels as it prevents disruption of blood flow, which could otherwise lead to complications such as edema. After accessing the vein, the next step is to locate the artery. Place sterile drapes under the intended region to elevate the area and make the vessels more prominent, which helps visualization and palpation of the artery. Then, gently circumferentially dissect the artery and place a vessel loop around it to facilitate control and exposure of the artery. When accessing the artery and vein, it is crucial to be cautious of nearby structures, especially nerves, as careless handling can result in nerve damage (**Figure 5**).

For the next step, the vein is clamped as distally as possible to ensure maximum length for anastomosis. The vein is then transected, with the distal end ligated with a silk tie to prevent any backflow. A vessel probe is then passed through the vein to dilate it as preparation for anastomosis. The vein is then flushed with a heparinized saline solution and clamped proximally to prevent thrombosis during the anastomotic process. This step also helps evaluate whether any obstruction or stenosis is present in the vein and to ensure that it will not twist as it mobilizes toward the artery. For the artery, a vessel clamp is placed proximally and distally to the planned anastomosis site. To note, the vessel clamp is positioned like the illustration below to help minimize the risk of injuring the posterior wall of the vessel. Arteriotomy is done with a diameter slightly smaller than the vein to ensure a sufficient anastomotic connection. The anastomosis is then completed in an end-to-side fashion, which is commonly used for AVF creation. One of the most critical aspects of this procedure is managing the heel and toe of the anastomosis, which are common points of access failure. The heel of the vein is typically positioned at the 12 o'clock

DOI: http://dx.doi.org/10.5772/intechopen.1011671

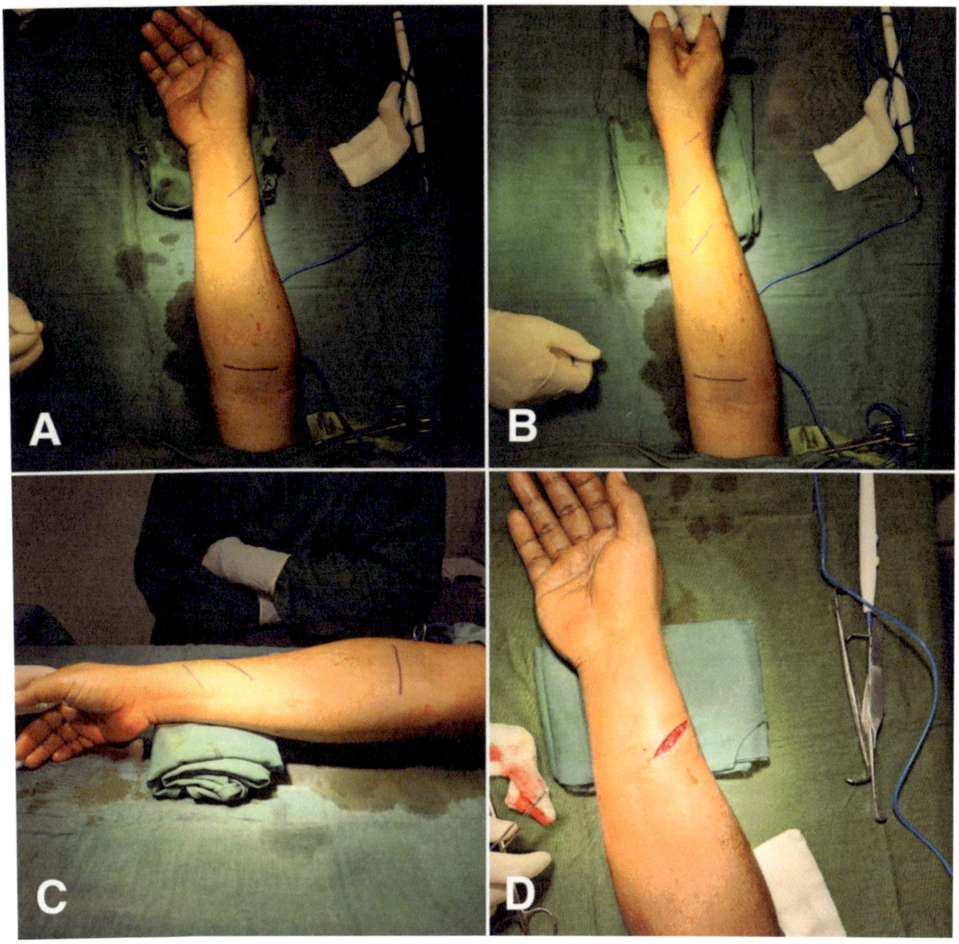

Figure 5.
Skin preparation and forearm positioning before AVF access creation. As shown in (A) and (B), incision sites may vary based on the intended vascular access target. To help identify the artery, a sterile drape is placed beneath the arm (C). For wrist access, a skin incision is made diagonally along the radial side (D).

position of the vein, which commonly will be sutured to the corresponding 12 o'clock position of the artery. However, this alignment may need to be adjusted depending on the anatomical distance and position between the vein and artery; thus, it is advisable to ensure that both vessels are not twisted during the process, as it may affect patency in the long term. There are two well-known continuous suturing techniques for creating the anastomosis: the parachute technique and the anchor technique. The parachute technique is more useful in the setting of smaller or deeper veins, as it allows for greater visualization of the anastomosis and a more controlled tension distribution. However, this technique carries an increased risk of potentially injuring the vessels, particularly in the structurally compromised vessels, such as those affected by atherosclerosis or thin venous walls. Conversely, the anchor technique is more suitable for larger and more superficial veins. Suturing can be done in an in-out or forehand approach, with the in-out suture being more helpful for ensuring proper alignment of the vessels. Suture methods preserving intimal alignment and minimizing endothelial trauma are critical for reducing long-term vascular complications, such as thrombosis and atherosclerosis. Studies by Mabrouk et al. [43] and Vyahalkar et al. [44] have compared the parachute and anchor anastomotic suturing techniques, with both studies indicating that the parachute technique is associated with better technical success and short-term primary patency outcome. Once the anastomotic sutures are in place, before tightening them, remove the proximal artery clamp to allow for deairing. Finally, all clamps are removed, and the anastomosis is thoroughly checked for any signs of leakage to ensure the integrity of the connection (**Figure 6**).

In basilic vein transposition, the anastomotic technique basically adheres to the same principles as those used in standard AVF access creation, as previously described. The first critical aspect is the identification of anatomical landmarks in the brachial region. Meticulous dissection of the brachial artery and vein is essential to avoid injury to adjacent neural structures, particularly the median and ulnar nerves. Based on our clinical experience, we recommend a combination of blunt and sharp dissection techniques rather than electrocautery, as thermal energy can easily damage surrounding nerves. Second, prior to clamping the artery or vein, it is advisable to administer heparin at a dose of 100 IU/kg to minimize the risk of thrombus formation, especially given the prolonged operative time required for basilic vein transposition. This anticoagulation step is equally important in AVG placement for the same rationale. Lastly, during the tunneling process, after dissection of the basilic vein, intraluminal distention using a heparinized saline solution should be performed to evaluate for the presence of stenosis. If no narrowing is detected, vein tunneling can be done while maintaining continuous saline distension, following the same principle applied in AVF placement to ensure vein patency and facilitate successful anastomosis.

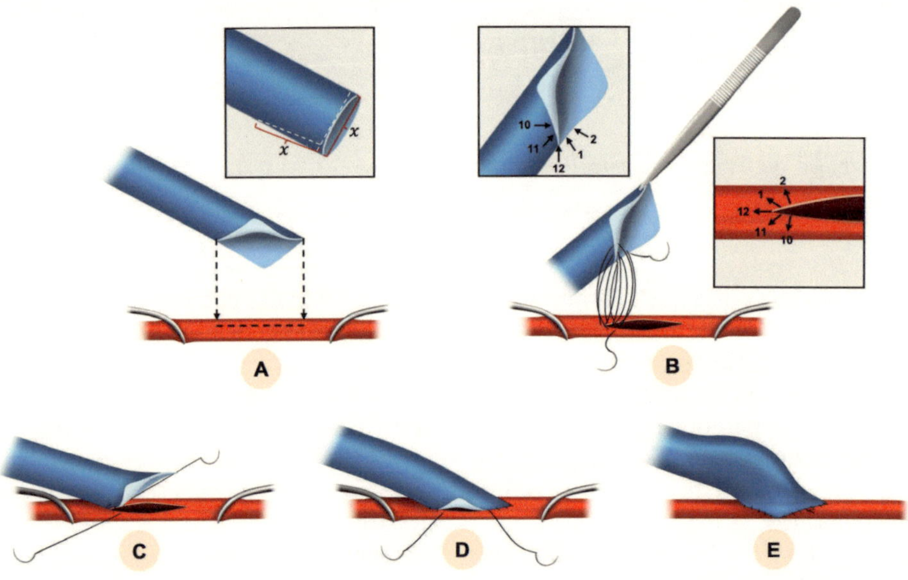

Figure 6.
Anastomosis technique. Venotomy is performed with an incision approximately twice the diameter of the original vein, followed by arteriotomy, which is made slightly smaller than the vein (A). The 12 o'clock position of the vein is commonly sutured to the 12 o'clock position of the artery, although this may vary depending on the alignment of the vessels (B). The vessels are then sutured using either the parachute or anchor technique (C-D). If anastomosis is completed, ensure the vein is adequately dilated and check for any signs of leakage (E).

DOI: http://dx.doi.org/10.5772/intechopen.1011671

Next, in the AVG access creation utilizing SVG conduit, thorough preoperative evaluation of both the SVG and the target venous outflow site using DUS is essential. It is crucial that the diameters of the SVG and the target vein are comparable, as significant size discrepancies may induce turbulent flow, increasing the risk of thrombosis and subsequent stenosis. Moreover, it is important to consider the presence of valves within the SVG. Proper orientation of the proximal and distal ends is necessary to ensure unobstructed flow and avoid hemodynamic compromise. The anastomosis and tunneling principles are similar to those applied in AVF creation and basilic vein transposition. However, particular caution is necessary when anastomosing the graft to a native vein, as these recipient veins often have thin walls and are located deeper within the tissue, thus presenting a technical challenge during anastomosis. Surgical precision and meticulous handling are therefore essential to minimize the risk of complications and ensure successful graft function.

Acknowledgements

The authors wish to thank the other members of the Cardiac, Thoracic, and Vascular Surgery department at Gadjah Mada University for their help throughout the course of this work.

Conflict of interest

The authors declare no conflict of interest.

Appendices and nomenclature

Abbreviations

CKD	chronic kidney disease
ESKD	end-stage kidney disease
KRT	kidney replacement therapy
HD	hemodialysis
CVC	central venous catheter
AVF	arteriovenous fistula
AVG	arteriovenous graft
GFR	glomerular filtration rate
KDOQI	kidney disease outcomes quality initiative
DUS	duplex ultrasound
CTA	computed tomography angiography
DSA	digital subtraction angiography
DSV	digital subtraction venography
MRA	magnetic resonance angiography
NTDCs	nontunneled dialysis catheters
TDCs	tunneled dialysis catheters
DAPT	dual antiplatelet therapy
SAPT	single antiplatelet therapy
ePTFE	expanded polytetrafluoroethylene
APT	antiplatelet therapy

Author details

Yunanto Kurnia[1*], Trianingsih[2] and Maura Andini Setiabudi[3]

1 Division of Cardiothoracic and Vascular Surgery, Department of Surgery, Faculty of Medicine, Public Health and Nursing, Universitas Gadjah Mada, Dr. Sardjito General Hospital, Yogyakarta, Indonesia

2 Department of Radiology, Faculty of Medicine, Public Health and Nursing, Universitas Gadjah Mada, Dr. Sardjito General Hospital, Yogyakarta, Indonesia

3 Faculty of Medicine, Public Health and Nursing, Universitas Gadjah Mada, Yogyakarta, Indonesia

*Address all correspondence to: yunantokurnia@ugm.ac.id

IntechOpen

© 2025 The Author(s). Licensee IntechOpen. This chapter is distributed under the terms of the Creative Commons Attribution License (http://creativecommons.org/licenses/by/4.0), which permits unrestricted use, distribution, and reproduction in any medium, provided the original work is properly cited.

References

[1] Kovesdy CP. Epidemiology of chronic kidney disease: An update 2022. Kidney International. Supplement. 2022;**12**(1):7-11. DOI: 10.1016/j.kisu.2021.11.003

[2] Lok CE, Huber TS, Lee T, Shenoy S, Yevzlin AS, Abreo K, et al. KDOQI clinical practice guideline for vascular access: 2019 update. American Journal of Kidney Diseases. 2020;**75**(4):S1-S164. DOI: 10.1053/j.ajkd.2019.12.001

[3] Flythe JE, Watnick S. Dialysis for chronic kidney failure: A review. JAMA. 2020;**332**(18):1559-1573. Available from: http://www.ncbi.nlm.nih.gov/pubmed/39356511

[4] Yoshida M, Doi S, Nakashima A, Kyuden Y, Kawai T, Kawaoka K, et al. Different risk factors are associated with vascular access patency after construction and percutaneous transluminal angioplasty in patients starting hemodialysis. The Journal of Vascular Access. 2021;**22**(5):707-715

[5] Garcia-Lopez AE, Sánchez R, Vesga JI, Sanabria RM. Factors associated with hemodialysis vascular access failure: A retrospective study in Colombia. Revista Colombiana de Nefrología. 2023;**10**(1):1-14

[6] Long J, Chen H, Huang Q, Chen X, Ellis RJ, Zanoli L, et al. Analysis of risk factors for late arteriovenous fistula failure and patency rates after angioplasty in hemodialysis patients: A retrospective cohort study. Translational Andrology and Urology. 2024;**13**(2):209-217

[7] De Pinho NA, Coscas R, Metzger M, Labeeuw M, Ayav C, Jacquelinet C, et al. Predictors of nonfunctional arteriovenous access at hemodialysis initiation and timing of access creation: A registry-based study. PLoS One. 2017;**12**(7):1-15

[8] Richarz S, Isaak A, Aschwanden M, Partovi S, Staub D. Pre-procedure imaging planning for dialysis access in patients with end-stage renal disease using ultrasound and upper extremity computed tomography angiography: A narrative review. Cardiovascular Diagnosis and Therapy. 2023;**13**(1):122-132

[9] Sohail MA, Vachharajani TJ, Anvari E. Central venous catheters for hemodialysis—The myth and the evidence. Kidney International Reports. 2021;**6**(12):2958-2968. DOI: 10.1016/j.ekir.2021.09.009

[10] Engstrom BI, Horvath JJ, Stewart JK, Sydnor RH, Miller MJ, Smith TP, et al. Tunneled internal jugular hemodialysis catheters: Impact of laterality and tip position on catheter dysfunction and infection rates. Journal of Vascular and Interventional Radiology. 2013;**24**(9):1295-1302. DOI: 10.1016/j.jvir.2013.05.035

[11] Shingarev R, Barker-Finkel J, Allon M. Association of hemodialysis central venous catheter use with ipsilateral arteriovenous vascular access survival. American Journal of Kidney Diseases. 2012;**60**(6):983-989

[12] Echefu G, Stowe I, Lukan A, Sharma G, Basu-Ray I, Guidry L, et al. Central vein stenosis in hemodialysis vascular access: Clinical manifestations and contemporary management strategies. Frontiers in Nephrology. 2023;**3**(November):1-13

[13] Parienti JJ, Thirion M, Mégarbane B, Souweine B, Ouchikhe A, Polito A, et al.

Femoral vs jugular venous catheterization and risk of nosocomial events in adults. A Randomized Controlled Trial. JAMA. 2008;**299**(20):2413-2422

[14] Marik PE, Flemmer M, Harrison W. The risk of catheter-related bloodstream infection with femoral venous catheters as compared to subclavian and internal jugular venous catheters: A systematic review of the literature and meta-analysis. Critical Care Medicine. 2012;**40**(8):2479-2485

[15] Sakuraya M, Okano H, Yoshihiro S, Niida S, Kimura K. Insertion site of central venous catheter among hospitalized adult patients: A systematic review and network meta-analysis. Frontiers in Medicine. 2022;**9**

[16] Manov JJ, Mohan PP, Vazquez-Padron R. Arteriovenous fistulas for hemodialysis: Brief review and current problems. The Journal of Vascular Access. 2022;**23**(5):839-846

[17] Arasu R, Jegatheesan D, Sivakumaran Y. Overview of hemodialysis access and assessment. Canadian Family Physician. 2022;**68**(8):577-582

[18] Siddiqui MA, Ashraff S, Carline T. Maturation of arteriovenous fistula: Analysis of key factors. Kidney Research and Clinical Practice. 2017;**36**(4):318-328

[19] Aljarrah Q, Al Bakkar L, Bakkar S, Abou-Foul AK, Allouh MZ. Perioperative vascular access mapping in patients with hemodialysis: A comparative study of access navigation and selection in Jordan. Vascular Health and Risk Management. 2024;**20**(September):421-434

[20] Siddiqui MA, Ashraff S, Santos D, Rush R, Carline T, Raza Z. Predictive parameters of arteriovenous fistula maturation in patients with end-stage renal disease. Kidney Research and Clinical Practice. 2018;**37**(3):277-286

[21] Marques, da Silva B, Fernandes J, Oliveira J, Silva H, Fortes A, Lopes JA, et al. Preoperative assessment for vascular access: Vascular mapping and handgrip strength. The Journal of Vascular Access. 2024;**25**(5):1627-1634

[22] Kakkos SK, Kaplanis N, Papachristou EC, Papadoulas SI, Lampropoulos GC, Tsolakis IA, et al. The significance of inflow artery and tourniquet derived cephalic vein diameters on predicting successful use and patency of arteriovenous fistulas for haemodialysis. European Journal of Vascular and Endovascular Surgery. 2017;**53**(6):870-878. DOI: 10.1016/j.ejvs.2017.02.006

[23] Feng R, Wang S, Yu J, Zheng X, Chen W, Wang X, et al. The feasibility and efficiency for constructing arteriovenous fistula with <2 mm vein—A systematic review and meta-analysis. Frontiers in Cardiovascular Medicine. 2023;**10**(September):1-8

[24] Kordzadeh A, Mouhsen MIMM, Prionidis I, Francesconi M, Inston N. Vessel diameter and radiocephalic arteriovenous fistula: A meta-analysis and Markov model. Journal of Vascular Surgery. 2025;**82**(1):286-294. DOI: 10.1016/j.jvs.2025.02.031

[25] Oprea A, Molnar A, Vlăduțiu D, Scridon T, Trifan C, Săcui D, et al. Correlation between preoperative vein and artery diameters and arteriovenous fistula outcome in patients with end-stage renal disease. Medicine and Pharmacy Reports. 2018;**91**(4):399-407

[26] Nantakool S, Rerkasem K, Reanpang T, Worraphan S,

Prasannarong M. A systematic review with meta-analysis of the effects of arm exercise training programs on arteriovenous fistula maturation among people with chronic kidney disease. Hemodialysis International. 2020;**24**(4):439-453

[27] Pirozzi N, Mancianti N, Scrivano J, Fazzari L, Pirozzi R, Tozzi M. Monitoring the patient following radio-cephalic arteriovenous fistula creation: Current perspectives. Vascular Health and Risk Management. 2021;**17**:111-121

[28] Alqahtani SS, Aljaber FK, Alsuwailem BY, Almashouq YA, Bander G. Dialysis access-associated steal syndrome in high-risk patients undergoing surgery for hemodialysis access: A systematic review and meta-analysis of preventive operative techniques. Cureus. 2023;**15**(11):e498612

[29] Lin R, Qian J, He H, Zhao Y, Lv J, Peng J, et al. Correlation between preoperative Doppler ultrasonographyassessed specific accessory cephalic vein diameter-cephalic vein diameter ratio (r) and early dysfunction of radial artery-cephalic vein arteriovenous fistula: A single-center cross-sectional study. Quantitative Imaging in Medicine and Surgery. 2023;**13**(9):5796-5802

[30] Al-Jaishi AA, Liu AR, Lok CE, Zhang JC, Moist LM. Complications of the arteriovenous fistula: A systematic review. Journal of the American Society of Nephrology. 2017;**28**(6):1839-1850

[31] Twine CP, Kakkos SK, Aboyans V, Baumgartner I, Behrendt CA, Bellmunt-Montoya S, et al. Editor's choice—European Society for Vascular Surgery (ESVS) 2023 clinical practice guidelines on antithrombotic therapy for vascular diseases. European Journal of Vascular and Endovascular Surgery. 2023;**65**(5):627-689

[32] Park HS, Kim WJ, Kim YK, Kim HW, Choi BS, Park CW, et al. Comparison of outcomes with arteriovenous fistula and arteriovenous graft for vascular access in hemodialysis: A prospective cohort study. American Journal of Nephrology. 2016;**43**(2):120-128

[33] Li J, Lu H, Xie Z, Li Q, Shi H. Outcomes of arteriovenous graft vs. fistula for haemodialysis access in the elderly: A systematic review and meta-analysis. Experimental and Therapeutic Medicine. 2023;**26**(2):399

[34] Wuamett JC, Glickman MH. Arteriovenous graft configuration in hemodialysis: Does it matter? The Journal of Vascular Access. 2015;**16**(Suppl. 9): S78-S81

[35] Mousa AY, Patterson W, Abu-Halimah S, Hass SM, Alhalbouni S, Sadek BT, et al. Patency in arteriovenous grafts in hemodialysis patients. Vascular and Endovascular Surgery. 2013;**47**(6):438-443

[36] Berardinelli L. Grafts and graft materials as vascular substitutes for haemodialysis access construction. European Journal of Vascular and Endovascular Surgery. 2006;**32**(2):203-211

[37] Yousef AA, Abdelwahab MB, EA AEL-M, Waly MA. Alternative grafts for brachioaxillary hemodialysis access: Saphenous vein versus synthetic graft (comparative study). Benha Journal of Applied Sciences. 2020;**5**(4):1-8

[38] Halbert RJ, Nicholson G, Nordyke RJ, Pilgrim A, Niklason L. Patency of ePTFE arteriovenous graft placements in hemodialysis patients: Systematic literature review and meta-analysis. Kidney360. 2020;**1**(12):1437-1446

[39] Ebertz DP, Bose S, De Valle A, Locham S, Malas Malas MB, Smeds MR. Single or dual antiplatelet therapy improves one-year arteriovenous graft patency and overall survival. Annals of Vascular Surgery. 2024;**100**(February):266-267

[40] Locham S, Beaulieu RJ, Dakour-Aridi H, Nejim B, Malas MB. Role of antiplatelet therapy in the durability of hemodialysis access. Journal of Nephrology. 2018;**31**(4):603-611. DOI: 10.1007/s40620-018-0490-6

[41] Yen CC, Tu HP, Lin TC, Li KY, Chen SC. Routine clinic surveillance on arteriovenous graft patency in hemodialysis patients with previous access complications. International Journal of Medical Sciences. 2025;**22**(5):1064-1071

[42] El-Kenany MAAA, Ghalwash IT, MAEH AER. Management of complications of arteriovenous grafts in patients with chronic renal failure. Egyptian Journal of Hospital Medicine. 2018;**72**(5):4505-4508

[43] Mabrouk M, Atta I, Fouda A, Ismail K, Ismail T, Gawish R, et al. Anchor versus parachute suturing technique in arteriovenous fistula creation for hemodialysis. Vascular. 2024;**13**:1-10

[44] Vyahalkar SV, Chaudhari AE, Binnani PG, Kulkarni AV, Nagarik AP, Jawade KK, et al. Comparative study of the effects of two suturing techniques of end-to-side arteriovenous anastomosis on early outcomes of radio-cephalic fistulas. Indian Journal of Vascular and Endovascular Surgery. 2021;**8**(Suppl. 2): S130-S136